MANAGEMENT OF

Respiratory Tract
Infections

MANAGEMENT OF

Respiratory Tract Infections

JOHN G. BARTLETT, M.D.

Professor of Medicine
Chief, Division of Infectious Diseases
John Hopkins University School of Medicine
Baltimore, Maryland

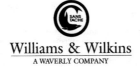

Williams & Wilkins
A WAVERLY COMPANY

BALTIMORE • PHILADELPHIA • LONDON • PARIS • BANGKOK
BUENOS AIRES • HONG KONG • MUNICH • SYDNEY • TOKYO • WROCLAW

Editor: Jonathan W. Pine, Jr.
Managing Editor: Molly L. Mullen
Production Coordinator: Marette D.
Magargle-Smith

Typesetter: Graphic World, Inc.
Printer & Binder: Vicks Lithograph &
Printing

Accurate indications, adverse reactions and dosage schedules for drugs are provided
in this book, but it is possible that they may change. The reader is urged to review the
package information data of the manufacturers of the medications mentioned.

Printed in the United States of America

Library of Congress Cataloging-in-Publication Data

Bartlett. John G.
    Management of respiratory tract infections / John G. Bartlett.
        p.   cm.
    Includes index.
    ISBN 0–683–30236–1
    1.   Respiratory infections.   I. Title.
    [DNLM: 1.   Respiratory Tract Infections.   WF 140 B289m 1997]
RC740.B37   1997
616.2—dc21
DNLM/DLC   97–13539
for Library of Congress   CIP

*The publishers have made every effort to trace the copyright holders for borrowed
material. If they have inadvertently overlooked any, they will be pleased to make
the necessary arrangements at the first opportunity.*

To purchase additional copies of this book, call our customer service department at
(800) 638-0672 or fax orders to **(800) 447-8438.** For other book services, including chapter reprints and large quantity sales, ask for the Special Sales department.

Canadian customers should call **(800) 268-4178,** or fax **(905) 470-6780.** For all
other calls originating outside of the United States, please call **(410) 528-4223** or
fax us at **(410) 528-8550.**

Visit Williams & Wilkins on the Internet: http://www.wwilkins.com or contact
our customer service department at **custserv@wwilkins.com.** Williams & Wilkins
customer service representatives are available from 8:30 am to 6:00 pm, EST,
Monday through Friday, for telephone access.

                                                                                97 98 99 00
                                                                    1 2 3 4 5 6 7 8 9 10

Preface

Respiratory tract infections are both common and important. In the United States and in the world, lower respiratory tract infections are the most common cause of death due to infectious disease. Upper respiratory tract infections are rarely lethal, but they are the source of extraordinary morbidity. Virtually everyone has upper respiratory tract infections. The total economic burden for the common cold is estimated at $2 billion per year in the United States.

Respiratory tract infections are also the source of most antibiotic use. Pharmaceutical industry research indicates that respiratory tract infections account for two-thirds of all antibiotic prescriptions. The good news is that this has had a favorable major impact on mortality rates—the "pneumococcus," for example, is no longer "captain of the men of death." On the other hand, respiratory tract infections are also the source of most antibiotic abuse, which contributes substantially to the problem of resistance. Paradoxically, the progress made in dealing with the pneumococcus, for example, is now associated with an unanticipated global explosion of penicillin resistance that has made treatment decisions suddenly complex.

The goal of this book is to deal with the issues related to repiratory tract infections. It is a clinically oriented book intended for practitioners, especially those in primary care. An attempt has been made to synthesize complex data from diverse sources to provide a practical management approach to common clinical conditions. It is hoped that the emphasis on microbiology will reverse the escalating trend toward benign neglect of gumshoe microbiology in an era of managed care, outsourcing of laboratory studies, and of a consuming fetish for cost reduction. A second common theme concerns recommendations for antibiotics, with an effort to strike an appropriate balance that recognizes not only the extremes when these drugs are clearly indicated or not indicated, but also the relatively large gray zone where potential benefits are real but modest and likelihood of abuse is great.

John G. Bartlett, M.D.

Contents

CHAPTER 2

Acute and Chronic Cough Syndromes   118

CHAPTER 3

Common Cold   150

CHAPTER 4

Streptococcal Pharyngitis   172

CHAPTER 1

Pneumonia

John G. Bartlett

Overview

In the prepenicillin era, pneumonia caused by *Strepto-coccus pneumoniae* was popularly referred to by Osler as "captain of the men of death" and later as "the old man's friend," both in reference to the pivotal role of pneumo-cocci in morbidity and mortality. Since that time, there has been remarkable progress in the development of antibiotics to treat pneumonia, vaccines to prevent it; the introduction and expansion of multiple new antimicrobial agents, several new diagnostic techniques; and the critical development of respiratory support. The progress has been impressive, although pneumonia still represents a relatively common complication and substantial controversy remains concerning the use of diagnostic tests and recommendations for antibiotic therapy. The controversies are perhaps best highlighted by the fundamental differences in the guidelines for management published in 1993, which were based on consensus statements from two sophisticated groups: the American Thoracic Society (1) and the British Thoracic Society (2).

Pneumonia continues to play an important role in medicine. In the United States, it is the sixth leading cause of death and it is the most common cause of death due to infectious diseases (3). In the world, lower respiratory tract infections are the leading cause of death. This chapter reviews the current status of pneumonia to provide a rational approach to diagnosis and treatment. This information is restricted to adults.

DEFINITION

Pneumonia indicates inflammation of the lung parenchyma that is caused by a microbial agent. In many cases, the appellation is used to specify the clinical setting: community-acquired pneumonia (CAP), nursing home pneumonia, nosocomial pneumonia, pneumonia in the compromised host, aspiration pneumonia, and so forth. These terms are important because of differences in the likely microbial agent(s) in each case and, consequently, differences in antibiotic recommendations. Other classifications are based on disease tempo such as acute, subacute, or chronic pneumonia. Characteristic features may also be based on the observations with radiographic studies or computed tomography scans to characterize changes as lobar pneumonia, bronchopneumonia, interstitial pneumonia, lung abscess, hilar adenopathy, or pleural fluid. Finally, the pleural fluid may be characterized as transudate, exudate, or empyema.

DIAGNOSIS

Symptoms suggesting pneumonia include fever combined with respiratory complaints including cough, dyspnea, sputum production, and/or pleuritic chest pain. Patients with chronic pneumonia often complain of unintentional weight loss, chronic fatigue, and night sweats. Physical examination of patients with pneumonia shows fever in over 80%, crackles are heard on auscultation in 80%, and lobar consolidation is found in 15%–30%. The most important diagnostic test is the chest radiograph. Virtually all studies of pneumonia require the demonstration of an infiltrate accompanied by typical respiratory symptoms as diagnostic criteria, although clinicians will justifiably argue that rales ("crackles") or signs of consolidation on physical examination are equally compelling.

Chest radiograph. As noted, the diagnosis of pneumonia traditionally requires supporting evidence by a chest radiograph showing typical changes. There are four potential causes of a false-negative chest radiograph:

1. Dehydration: This is a rare cause of a false-negative chest radiograph and may actually represent an erroneous concept. Dogs challenged with *S. pneumoniae* show pulmonary infiltrates regardless of hydration status (4). In addition, dehydration does not account for the lack of an inflammatory reaction at other anatomic sites. Thus, dehydration, although commonly considered as a cause of false-negative chest radiographs, is weakly supported by available information.

2. Neutropenia: It is sometimes stated that patients with profound neutropenia will have false-negative radiographs based on the inability to generate an acute inflammatory reaction. This is theoretically conceivable, although the frequency is low.

3. Early course disease: Physicians in the prepenicillin era claim they could detect pneumonia by auscultation before the infiltrate was seen on chest radiograph. The allowable time for this delay is 24 hours. Again, this is rare and I have encountered only one typical case in the past 10 years.

4. *Pneumocystis carinii* pneumonia (PCP): *P. carinii* is the common exception in the acquired immunodeficiency syndrome (AIDS) epidemic. Most reports indicate 10%–20% of patients with PCP have a completely normal chest radiograph, and the frequency reaches 40% in some series (5).

The chest radiograph is considered pivotal for establishing the diagnosis of pneumonia owing to implications for management strategies. Most forms of pneumonia are treated with antimicrobial agents; most patients with typical respiratory complaints and negative chest radiographs have bronchitis, which is usually not treated with antimicrobial agents. It may be argued, especially in an era of cost constrains in managed care, that the chest radiograph is not cost-effective for the patient with cough and fever who is managed as an outpatient. In this case, the cost of an oral antibiotic is often substantially lower than that of the chest radiograph. Concerns with this tactic are the abuse of antibiotics (6) and the failure to document a potentially serious medical problem, including associated lesions.

False-positive radiograph results may also be problematic owing to the multitude of clinical conditions associated with pulmonary infiltrates, including pulmonary infarcts, congestive heart failure, carcinoma, Wegener's granulomatosis, sarcoidosis, interstitial lung disease, atelectasis, vasculitis, and so forth.

It is generally felt that chest radiographs do not distinguish bacterial versus nonbacterial infection. Nevertheless, some findings on chest radiograph often strongly support selected diagnoses (Table 1.1). The changes on chest radiograph also indicate the severity of the illness and serve as a guide for management decisions. Prognostic factors include the number of lobes involved and bilateral effusions (7).

Other laboratory tests. Diagnostic testing is usually limited in patients who are managed as outpatients. Potentially useful tests to consider are sputum on a glass slide for subsequent stain and microscopic examination, pulse oximetry, and complete blood count (CBC). The sputum sample for stain provides an opportunity for retrospective assessment of a specimen obtained prior to antimicrobial

Table 1.1
Chest Radiograph: Differential Diagnosis

Immunocompetent

Focal opacity

Streptococcus pneumoniae	*Chlamydia pneumoniae*
Hemophilus influenzae	*Staphylococcus aureus*
Mycoplasma pneumoniae	*Mycobacterium*
Legionella	*tuberculosis*

Interstitial/miliary

Viruses	*M. tuberculosis*
M. pneumoniae	Pathogenic fungi[a]

Hilar adenopathy ± segmental or interstitial infiltrate

Epstein Barr	*M. tuberculosis*
Tularemia	Pathogenic fungi[a]
C. psittaci	Atypical rubella
M. pneumoniae	

Cavitation

Anaerobes	Gram-negative bacilli
M. tuberculosis	*S. aureus*
Pathogenic fungi[a]	

[a]Pathogenic fungi: *Histoplasma capsulatum, Coccidioides immitis,* and *Blastomyces dermititidis.*

treatment. It is optimal to obtain the Gram stain interpretation prior to treatment, but many physicians in office practice do not have easy access to such information in a timely fashion. Other studies in outpatients may be done to determine the need for hospitalization. Tests that are advocated in patients who are hospitalized with pneumonia are summarized in Table 1.2. In general, these are done to determine the severity of illness, possible complications, and the status of underlying or associated conditions.

Table 1.2
Routine Tests in Hospitalized Patients with Community-Acquired Pneumonia

Chest radiograph
Arterial blood gas analysis
Complete blood count
Chemistry profile including renal and liver function tests and electrolytes
HIV serology (age 15–54 years)
Blood culture twice (before antibiotic treatment)
Sputum Gram stain and culture (before antibiotic treatment) ± AFB stain and culture, *Legionella* test (culture, DFA stain or urinary antigen), Mycoplasma IgM
Pleural fluid analysis (if present): WBC and differential, LDH, pH, protein, glucose, Gram stain, AFB stain, and culture for bacteria (aerobes and anaerobes) and mycobacteria

HIV, human immunodeficiency virus; AFB, acid-fast bacillus; DFA, WBC, white blood cell count; LDH, lactate dehydrogenase.

The complete blood count is considered standard. Anemia often indicates mycoplasma infection, chronic disease, or complicated pneumonia. The white blood count is generally not useful for distinguishing causative agents, although a count above 15,000/mL suggests bacterial infection, and counts below 3000/mL or above 25,000/mL appear to be prognostic indicators.

Human immunodeficiency virus (HIV) serology is often suggested for patients aged 15–54 years who are seriously ill with pneumonia (8). Many of these patients will deny the usual risk factors. One study from an urban center (Johns Hopkins Hospital) showed 35 of 385 patients (9%) admitted with CAP had previously unrecognized HIV infection (9). In the absence of the availability of serologic testing or a delay in reporting, the physician considering late-stage HIV infection should review the white blood count and differential diagnosis to determine if there is lymphopenia with an absolute lymphocyte count less than 1000/dL. This supports the possibility of HIV infection. A better test is the CD4 cell count, which is rarely lower than 200/mm^3 in any other condition.

Blood gas determination is an important prognostic indicator. Hypoxemia with a pO_2 of less than 60 mm Hg on room air represents a standard criterion for hospital admission and consideration for the intensive care unit (ICU) (10).

Pleural effusions are found in up to 30% of patients with CAP and many other forms of pulmonary infection as well. Thoracentesis should be done if there is a delay in resolution, a large collection of pleural effusions, or an unsettled diagnosis. Pleural fluid that is grossly purulent is diagnostic of empyema and requires drainage. Analysis of pleural fluid should include pH, glucose, protein, lactic dehydrogenase, white blood count, Gram stain, acid-fast bacillus (AFB) stain, and cultures for bacteria (aerobes and anaerobes), fungi, and mycobacteria. (Blood count and chemistries are unnecessary with purulent effusions.) A pH greater than 7.3 predicts response to antibiotic treatment; a pH less than 7.1 predicts the necessity for drainage (11). Meta-analysis of empyema reports suggest pleural fluid pH is the most useful test to determine effusions that require drainage (12).

ETIOLOGIC DIAGNOSIS

The diagnosis of pneumonia is fraught with great problems owing to the difficulty of getting uncontaminated specimens from the source of infection. The two major problems are the fact that any specimen that is contaminated by secretions from the upper airways is usually inconclusive and specimens from nearly all sources are unreliable for detection of common pathogens if antibiotic treatment has been initiated. In general, a confirmed etiologic diagnosis requires one of the following:

1. Recovery of a likely pulmonary pathogen from an uncontaminated specimen source including blood, pleural

fluid, transtracheal aspirate, transthoracic aspirate or from a metastatic site of infection, such as meningitis or septic arthritis.

2. The detection of an organism that is a likely pulmonary pathogen and does not colonize the upper or lower airways in the absence of disease: *Mycobacterium tuberculosis, Legionella,* pathogenic fungi, *(Histoplasma capsulatum, Coccidioides immitis, Blastomyces dermatitis, Cryptococcus neoformans), Strongyloides,* influenza virus, respiratory syncytial virus (RSV), *Hantavirus,* adenovirus, coxsackie virus, *Pneumocystis carinii,* and *Toxoplasma gondii. M. pneumoniae* and *Chlamydia pneumoniae* have occasionally been recovered from healthy adults, but only rarely.

3. Serologic tests that are considered relatively specific based on arbitrary criteria for the timing and titer. However, there are many serologic criteria for which there is no consensus regarding the technique for study; some assays are nonspecific owing to antigenic cross-reactions and some show serologic reactions that represent nonspecific antigenic stimuli. The greatest problem is the temporal requirement for the serologic rise in titer necessary for a confirmed diagnosis.

In reality, no causative agent is clearly identified by any of these three criteria in a large majority of cases. The result is that the physician is usually required to interpret the results of less definitive studies such as expectorated sputum Gram stain and culture. Alternative specimen sources such as transtracheal aspiration, transthoracic needle aspiration, or bronchoscopy, are usually reserved for cases that are unusual due to atypical presentation, severe disease, disease in a specific host setting, such as the compromised host, or in patients who fail to respond to treatment. In many cases, the diagnostic test of choice is specific to the microbial agent (Table 1.3).

Table 1.3
Pulmonary Infections: Specimens and Tests for Detection of Lower Respiratory Pathogens

Organism	Specimen	Microscopy	Culture	Serology*	Other
Bacteria Aerobic and facultatively anaerobic	Expectorated sputum, blood, TTA, empyema fluid, lung biopsy	Gram stain	X	—	
Anaerobic	TTA, empyema fluid	Gram stain	X	—	
Legionella sp	Sputum, lung biopsy, pleural fluid, TTA	FA (L. pneumophilia)	X	IFA, EIA	Urinary antigen (L. pneumophila grl)[a] PCR (experimental)
Nocardia sp	Expectorated sputum, TTA, bronchial washing, BAL fluid, tissue	Gram and modified carbol fuchsin stain	X	—	
Chlamydia sp	Nasopharyngeal swab	Negative	X[a]	CF for C. psittaci; MIF for C pneumoniae CF, EIA	PCR of throat swab for C. pneumoniae (experimental)

*CMV, cytomegalovirus; BAL, bronchoalveolar lavage; CF, complement fixation; CIE, counterimmunoelectrophoresis; DFA, direct fluorescent antibody; EIA, enzyme immunoassay; FA, florescent antibody stain; GMS, Gomori-methenamine stain; H&E, hematoxylin and eosin; ID, immunodiffusions; IFA, indirect fluorescent antibody; KOH, potassium hydroxide; LA;, MIF, microimmunofluorescence test; PCR, polymerase chain reaction; PPD, purified protein derivative; RSV, respiratory syncytial virus; TTA, transtracheal aspiration.

[a]Not offered by most laboratories.

(continued)

				Table 1.3 (continued)	

Organism	Specimen	Microscopy	Culture	Serology*	Other
Mycoplasma sp	Nasopharyngeal swab	Negative	X[a]		PCR[a] of throat swab (experimental)
Mycobacteria	Expectorated or induced sputum, TTA, bronchial washing, BAL fluid	Fluorochrome stain or carbol fuchsin	X	—	PPD, PCR (experimental)
Fungi					
Deep-seated					
Blastomyces sp	Expectorated or induced sputum, bronchial washing or biopsy, BAL fluid, tissue	KOH with phase contrast, GMS stain	X	CF, ID	Antigen assay of BAL, blood, urine (call 1-800-HISTO-DG)
Coccidiodes sp			X	CF, ID, LA	
Histoplasma sp			X	CF, ID	
Opportunistic					
Aspergillus sp	Lung biopsy	H&E, GMS stain	X	ID	CT scan
Candida sp	Lung biopsy	H&E, GMS stain	X	—	
Cryptococcus sp	Expectorated sputum, serum, transbronch bx or BAL	H&E, GMS stain Calcofluor white	X	—	Serum or BAL antigen assay
Zygomycetes	Expectorated sputum, tissue	H&E, GMS stain	X	—	

(continued)

Table 1.3 (continued)

Organism	Specimen	Microscopy	Culture	Serology*	Other
Viruses: influenza, paraflu, RSV, CMV	Nasal washings, naso-pharyngeal aspirate or swab, BAL fluid, lung biopsy	FA: influenza and RSV	X[a]	CF, EIA, LA, FA	CMV: shell viral culture, FA stain of BAL or bx Influenza–nasal swab for tissue culture; DFA stain RSV-FA stain
Hantavirus	Blood	Negative	—	Western blot for IgG and IgM[a]	PCR[a] (experimental) CBC—hemoconcentration, thrombocytopenia, leuko-cytosis, and immunoblasts
Pneumocystis sp	Induced sputum or bronchial brushings, washings, BAL fluid	Toluidine blue, Giemsa, FA, or GMS stain	—	—	
Coxiella burnetti					

Expectorated sputum. The diagnostic utility of expectorated sputum testing by Gram stain and culture has been debated for decades. In the late 1960s and early 1970s several studies showed the yield of *S. pneumoniae* in expectorated sputum culture from patients with bacteremic pneumococcal pneumonia was only about 50% (Table 1.4) (13–15). Additional studies showed that the frequency of false-positive cultures for this organism in the absence of respiratory disease approached 50% as well (16). The conclusion was that the usual specimen source used to detect *S. pneumoniae,* the most common identifiable agent of lower respiratory tract infections, was associated with both false-negative and false-positive results in about 50% of cases. This experience raised grave doubts regarding the diagnostic utility of expectorated sputum. Consequently, rather intensive efforts in the 1970s dealt more effectively with the issue of pathogen detection. Two tactics were adopted: The first was an attempt to obtain specimens that were not contaminated by the upper airway flora by utilizing transtracheal aspiration, transthoracic needle aspiration, or bronchoscopy aspirates. The second tactic was based on the philosophy that the only practical specimen to obtain was expectorated sputum, dealt and it was nec-

Table 1.4
Yield of *Streptococcus pneumoniae* in Cultures of Expectorated Sputum from Patients with Bacteremic Pneumococcal Pneumonia

Source	Sensitivity[a]
Rathbun HK (1967) (15)	31/69 (45%)
Fiala M (1969) (14)	11/25 (44%)
Barrett-Conner E (1970) (13)	25/48 (52%)

[a]Number with *S. pneumoniae* in expectorated sputum culture per number with pneumonia and *S. pneumoniae* in blood cultures.

essary to deal with the problem of contamination during passage through the upper airways by using wash procedures, quantitation of bacteria, and cytologic screening. From these studies, the only technique that has withstood the test of time and subsequently was incorporated into standard laboratory practice is cytologic screening of the expectorated sputum sample (Table 1.5) (17).

Most investigators now feel that expectorated sputum Gram stain and culture is worthwhile with the following caveats:

1. The specimen must be obtained before antibiotic treatment.

2. Good quality control efforts are needed in specimen procurement, expeditious transport to the laboratory, and proper processing. Delays in time from collection to incubation that exceed 2–5 hours are associated with deceptive results (18). (It might be noted that the high yield of *S. pneumoniae* in the prepenicillin era was largely ascribed to techniques that have subsequently become uncommon, such as plating on the ward, and the use of the Quellung stain and mouse inoculation). One of the explanations for the sharp decrease in the yield of *S. pneumoniae* at Johns Hopkins Hospital in the study done in 1991 (9) compared with the study done in 1971 (18% vs. 62%) is that the study with the high yield was done with prompt plating and incubation on the ward (19).

3. Cytologic screening is needed to demonstrate the presence of secretions from the lower airway with limited contamination from the upper airways. The original criteria were a low power examination (100×) showing more than 25 polymorphonuclear leukocytes per field and less than 10 epithelial cells/field (17). Subsequent modifications have been made and many laboratories have now adopted a criterion of less than 25 epithelial cells as a contingency for culture (20,21).

Table 1.5
Guidelines for Sputum Bacteriology

Specimen collection

Patient should rinse mouth before producing sputum

Specimen must be deep cough which should be purulent with minimal saliva

Induced sputum using inhalation of hypertonic saline is useful primarily in patients who are unable to produce an expectorated sample. Utility is established for detection of *Mycobacteria* in patients who cannot produce expectorated sputum and *Pneumocystis carinii.*

With suspected mycobacterial or fungal pneumonia, collect three morning specimens; a single specimen is adequate for conventional bacteria providing cytologic creening is adequate.

Transport

Expectorated sputum and respiratory secretions collected by other means should be transported and processed within 2–5 hours of collection (18).

Processing

A purulent portion of the sample is selected for stains and culture

Cytologic screening is done with Gram stain under low power magnification ($\times 100$) to determine the ratio of polymorphonuclear cells and squamous epithelial cells. Laboratories use different criteria to judge adequacy, but the classic study used a criterion of <10 squamous epithelial cells/low power field and >25 polymorphonuclear cells (17).

The smear is next examined under oil emersion ($\times 1000$). Sensitivity of the Gram stain is high, but specificity is low. Conversely, if typical lancet-shaped Gram-positive diplococci are seen or shown to be Quellung positive, the sensitivity is 50%, but specificity is high (24).

Exceptions are specimens for detection of *Mycobacteria* and *Legionella* that should not have cytologic screening.

4. Microbiology studies should include a Gram stain and culture, and the quality assurance program should demonstrate a correlation between the two. Most authorities conclude that Gram stains may show diagnostic information with good accuracy, although technical expertise is critical (22–25). The Johns Hopkins Hospital laboratory experience is that a likely microbial pathogen can be detected on Gram stain and culture in about 60% of expectorated sputum samples obtained prior to antibiotic treatment, and the organism suspected by Gram stain corresponds to the potential pathogen cultured in approximately 90% of cases (26). Prior antibiotic treatment decreases the likelihood of recovering a probable pathogen in 20%–30% of patients, the yield of fastidious bacteria *(Staphylococcus pneumoniae* and *Hemophilus influenzae)* is virtually nil and the probability of misleading resistant organisms such as Gram-negative bacilli (GNB) or *S. aureus* is high (9,26,27). Most laboratories report that 10%–70% of specimens are judged inadequate by cytologic criteria; the wide range reflects vagaries in the cytologic criteria (17,20,21) and in training of the professional staff who obtain specimens. With specimens that are suitable by cytologic criteria, a negative culture report is strong evidence that coliforms, pseudomonads, and *S. aureus* are not involved. This does not exclude fastidious organisms such as *S. pneumoniae* or *H. influenzae*.

5. Quantitation of bacteria improves diagnostic accuracy so that bacteria recovered in large concentrations are more likely to represent pathogens. This generally applies to bacterial infections at virtually any anatomic site including expectorated sputum (28) and broncho-

scopic aspirates (29). A practical alternative is the use of semiquantitative culture results of expectorated sputum. In general, growth in the second streak with more than 5–10 colonies constitutes "moderate growth."

Blood cultures. Interpretation of Gram stain and culture must be based on clinical correlations. Patients who are seriously ill, including most who are hospitalized, should have two blood cultures done prior to instituting antibiotic treatment. Although emphasis has been placed on obtaining specimens for microbiology studies prior to antibiotic treatment, this should not delay the initiation of antibiotic treatment, especially in patients who are seriously ill.

Pleural fluid. Patients with pleural effusions should have a diagnostic thoracentesis as discussed below (See pg 99).

SPECIMENS OBTAINED BY SPECIALIZED TECHNIQUES

The techniques, indications, complications, and diagnostic utility of transtracheal aspiration, transthoracic needle aspiration, and bronchoscopy specimens are summarized below (30–69).

Transtracheal aspiration. Transtracheal aspiration (TTA) was originally reported in 1958 (30) and subsequently became a popular procedure during the period from 1968 to about 1980. During this time there were many large series dealing with TTA in diverse settings, but there were also several reports of severe complications. The procedure is rarely done today, in part, because few are experienced in the technique (31).

Technique. The patient is placed in the supine position with the neck hyperextended. The notch between the lower border of the thyroid cartilage and cricoid cartilage is prepared and infiltrated with 1%–2% lidocaine with epinephrine (32). A 14-gauge needle of an intermediate-sized intracatheter is inserted through the cricoid membrane with open bevel facing forward, the needle is advanced a few millimeters into the trachea and angulated to ensure catheter passage in the caudal direction. The catheter is then passed to its full extent and the covering needle is withdrawn leaving the catheter in place. Aspiration is performed with a 20–30 mL syringe with a tight Luer lock attachment or with a suction apparatus. Often only a small amount of secretion enters the tubing, which should be transmitted immediately to the laboratory for processing.

Complications. Transtracheal aspiration is an unpleasant procedure for the patient due to the sensation of a foreign body in the lower airways. Complications can be divided in three categories: side effects of the needle puncture site, complications due to catheter placement in the lower airways, and vasovagal reactions. Major complications at the needle puncture site include bleeding, puncture of the posterior tracheal wall, cutaneous or paratracheal abscess, and subcutaneous emphysema. Serious complications, including fatalities, have been reported.

Diagnostic accuracy. Most of the published experience with TTA concerns patients with suspected bacterial infections of the lower airways, and here the results have been almost uniformly favorable providing the specimen is obtained before antibiotics are given (30–36). Our experience with 488 patients included 383 who satisfied clinical criteria for bacterial pneumonia; a likely pulmonary pathogen was recovered in 235 and 44 of 48 "false-negative" cultures were from patients who had previously received antibiotics (31). Restricting analysis to untreated patients, the true incidence of false-negative cultures was only 1%. There were 23 patients with bacteremic pneumococcal pneumonia and all 23 had positive TTAs for this organism. False-positive cultures occasionally occur in patients, primarily those with chronic bronchitis or bronchiectasis. Transtracheal aspirations in healthy medical students and others without chronic lung disease are usually sterile or show only nonpathogens in low numbers (35).

Contraindications. Severe hemoptysis, bleeding diathesis, and inability to cooperate with severe hypoxemia are contraindication to TTA. We generally require a platelet count exceeding 100,000/mL, a prothrombin time exceeding 60% of control, and a pO_2 exceeding 60 mm Hg with supplemented oxygen.

Indications. The usual indications for TTA are *a)* a suspected bacterial pathogen; *b)* alternative specimen sources using less invasive techniques are either inconclusive or not available; *c)* the severity of illness justifies the risk; *d)* technical expertise is available; *e)* antibiotics for this infection have not been given, and *f)* there are no patient contraindications (32). This technique has been used extensively to establish the diagnosis of anaerobic bacterial infections of the lower airways (36–38).

Transthoracic needle aspiration. The most extensive experience with transthoracic needle aspiration (TTNA) was in the prepenicillin era when the major indication for it was recovery of *S. pneumoniae* to provide the necessary information for administration of type-specific antisera, which was the only therapy available at the time (39). More recently, TTNA has been used primarily for cytologic evaluation of suspected malignancies and in occasional patients for a microbiologic diagnosis.

Technique. The area of involvement is determined by chest radiograph or computerized tomography (CT) scan and the site for needle introduction is identified with cutaneous markers, fluoroscopy, or with CT scan (40). The midaxillary line is the usual site of aspiration in patients with diffuse lung lesions. To assure proper needle placement, focal lesions require imaging guidance by biplane fluoroscopy, ultrasound, or computerized tomography. The local area is prepared and local anesthesia given. The procedure may be performed with a No. 18–22 gauge thin-walled spinal needle attached to a tight fitting 10–30 mL locking syringe or the thin No. 25 gauge needle that some prefer to reduce trauma. The needle is inserted during suspended respiration and the aspiration is made by negative pressure during slow withdrawal. The alternative technique is to install fluids such as saline or broth with suction aspiration. A postprocedure chest radiograph should be obtained several hours after completion to detect possible pneumothorax.

Complications. The most frequent complication is pneumothorax, which is noted in 20%–30%, but which is sufficiently severe to require chest tube drainage in 1%–10% (41). About 3%–10% of patients have hemoptysis during the procedure which is usually transient and self-limited. A rare, but potentially serious complication is air embolism. Herman and Hessel reported their results from a survey of 105 institutions with TTNA used in 1562 patients which showed death in 0.1%, major hemorrhage in 0.2%, and pneumothorax requiring a chest tube in 7% (42).

Diagnostic accuracy. A review of 19 reported series showed variable results (41). The diagnostic yield in patients with suspected bacterial pneumonia is reported at 35%–50%. Perhaps the most accurate definition of the rate of false-negative cultures is the experience with 211 patients with bacteremic pneumococcal pneumonia that showed positive results for this organism in 165 (78%) (39). The presumed explanation for false-negative results is improper needle placement, nonviable organisms, or involvement by organisms that cannot be routinely cultured, such as viruses and *Mycoplasma* and *Chlamydia*.

Contraindications. The major contraindications to TTNA use are bullous pulmonary disease in the region to be aspirated, requirement for mechanical ventilatory assistance, vascular lesions, and severe bleeding diathesis that cannot be corrected. Relative contraindications include localized lesions adjacent to major vessels, uncontrollable coughing, inability of the patient to cooperate, pulmonary hypertension, suspected Echinococcus cysts, and severe hypoxemia. Pneumothorax is the most common complication and patients with inadequate pulmonary reserve to tolerate a significant pneumothorax should not have this procedure.

Indications. The major indications for TTNA according to the American Thoracic Society are for the diagnosis of *a)* solitary nodules and masses, *b)* mediastinal and hilar masses, *c)* metastatic disease, *d)* chest wall invasion in lung cancer, and *e)* pulmonary infections and pulmonary nodules or air space consolidation (43). In adults, the major use has been for immunocompromised hosts or patients with atypical presentations in which the usual diagnostic specimen sources are either contraindicated or negative.

Bronchoscopy specimens. Bronchoscopy was developed in the late 1930s and fiberoptic techniques were introduced in the late 1960s, making it an attractive method to obtain specimens more directly from the lower airways to *a)* detect *M. tuberculosis* in patients without expectorated sputum; *b)* detect *P. carinii; c)* obtain cultures for "traditional" pulmonary pathogens, and *d)* detect diseases that require histology or cytopathology (41). Cultures of secretions obtained by suction aspiration through the inner channel for "conventional bacteria" are really no better than expectorated sputum (44). The reason is that the inner channel becomes filled with saliva during passage through the upper airways. This can be demonstrated by painting the posterior pharynx with methylene blue; the subsequent bronchoscopic aspirate is invariably blue in color and yields large concentrations of salivary bacteria.

Technique for detecting selected microbes. Detecting selected microbes refers to the use of bronchoscopy to obtain organisms from the lower airways that do not colonize the upper airways and consequently do not represent problems for interpretation. The most common are *M. tuberculosis,* and *P. carinii,* but it also applies to pathogenic fungi, *Legionella,* and most viruses. The yield for these pathogens is magnified by the use of multiple specimens including fixed-tissue specimens, touch imprints of tissue from transbronchial biopsy, bronchial lavage, and brush biopsies. For bronchoalveolar lavage (BAL), 20 mL of saline is added to the suction apparatus with a three-way stopcock; it is instilled and then aspirated using a vacuum of 50–100 mm Hg to collect the lavage fluid (45). This is repeated five times for a total installation of 100 mL and expected return of 40–70 mL. Aliquots of the fluid are then inoculated into appropriate media for recovery of microbes and the remaining fluid is useful for cytocentrifuge preparations using Gram stain for bacteria, the direct fluorescent antibody (DFA) stain for *Legionella,* acid-fast stain, and Gomori's methenamine silver stain for fungi and *P. carinii.*

Diagnostic yield. The diagnostic yield with *P. carinii* in patients with AIDS is over 95% (46). The *M. tuberculosis* yield is up to 94%, but lower rates are found by some (47). Many authorities feel that the yield of mycobacteria with expectorated sputum is at least as high or higher making bronchoscopy a preferred diagnostic test only if there is no expectorated sample. It should be noted that investigators using the Jackson bronchoscope in the 1950s and 1960s often called attention to the superior yield of the "post bronchoscopy specimen" in reference to the specimen collected after the procedure was over. A concern for the specimen obtained during the procedure was the large amount of lidocaine in the specimen because it has antibacterial properties. Nevertheless, this concern is unsubstantiated according to in vitro assays designed to simulate the routine technique (48). An advantage of bronchoscopy in some patients is the option of a transbronchial biopsy, which is especially attractive when focal lesions are within reach of the bronchoscope or when the differential diagnosis includes conditions that require histology such as cancer, interstitial lung disease, lymphocytic interstitial pneumonitis, or lymphoma.

Technique for detecting "conventional bacteria". Specimens collected by suction aspiration through the inner channel and processed with the usual microbiologic techniques represent no advantage over expectorated sputum or endotracheal tube aspiration. The problem is that the inner channel of the bronchoscope is invariably contaminated by saliva during passage through the upper airways. Alternative techniques that are now used extensively to improve the validity of bronchoscopy specimens include *a)* protected double-lumen brush catheter combined with quantitative culture (49–52); *b)* BAL with quantitative culture (52,53); and *c)* single brush catheter with quantitative culture (54). All three techniques require quantitative culture based on the assumption that bacterial pathogens are invariably present in concentrations exceeding 10^5/mL at the infected site and contaminants or colonizing bacteria are found in lower concentrations. (These general principles apply to bacterial infections at virtually any anatomic site) (55).

The techniques described for detecting conventional bacteria require a commitment by the bronchoscopist to follow rather precise methodology in obtaining the specimen and commitment by the microbiologist in performing quantitative cultures.

The patient is premedicated with atropine 30–60 minutes before the procedure and then with topical anesthesia using nebulized lidocaine (without preservative) (41,50,51). With the "double catheter protected swab" method, the bronchoscope is introduced and the catheter is inserted through the channel to the bronchoscope tip. The inner cannula is advanced to discharge the distal polyethylene glycol plug, and the inner channel is then advanced to the area of purulent collections. The brush is advanced to obtain secretions, then retracted, and the entire catheter system removed. The brush is used to prepare slides for Gram stain and any special stains, and the brush is then severed for placement into a transport vial containing 1 mL of sterile lactated Ringer's solution. In the laboratory, the vial is vortexed, and then a 0.1 mL aliquot is inoculated onto appropriate media; two successive 100 times dilutions are made so that the final dilutions are 10^{-1}, 10^{-3}, and 10^{-5}. Studies of brush specimens indicate that the volume of secretions on the brush vary from 0.01 to 0.001 mL so that growth at 10^{-3} dilutions represents 10^5 or 10^6 bacteria/milliliter (49). The single catheter device uses the same principles, but assumes that the quantitation is adequate to nullify the contamination that invariably occurs with catheter passage through the inner channel (52). With BAL, the specimens are transported and processed in a similar fashion, but there is disagreement about the threshold concentration considered "significant"; most consider 10^3 or 10^4/mL to be significant (52,53).

Accuracy. The validity of the double-lumen catheter with a distal occluding plug was demonstrated with in vitro tests using various catheter designs to sample a marker organism (pigmented *Serratia* sp.) after passage through a fiberoptic bronchoscope that had an inner channel filled with saliva (29). In vivo tests were then done by using this catheter in healthy controls (the investigators) and patients with infections or other lung problems. Extensive studies of the brush catheter by others and studies of BAL processed with quantitative culture have shown generally good results with minor exceptions (49,56–61). Nearly all who have reported poor correlations also report major departures from the techniques described above. The largest report concerns 172 patients; 75 of 78 (96%) patients with suspected bacterial pneumonia had a likely pathogen recovered in significant concentrations compared with only

2 of 35 control patients with alternative diagnoses (56). This report included 13 patients with bacteremic pneumonia and 12 of these had the blood culture isolate recovered in the bronchoscopy specimen. A similar high diagnostic yield is noted with Gram stain using the brush catheter specimen or centrifuged BAL (57).

Risks. Retrospective surveys of over 72,000 fiberoptic bronchoscopies showed 13 deaths (0.015%); the major risk is severe cardiovascular disease (62). There were also 41 life-threatening reactions ascribed to anesthesia and 2 deaths ascribed to hemorrhage following forceps biopsy. The transbronchial biopsy magnifies the risk substantially with a 5% risk of pneumothorax and 2%–3% risk of bleeding. Pereira, et al. noted a 16% incidence of transient fever and new pulmonary infiltrates in 6% of patients undergoing bronchoscopy (63). Others have found virtually no cases of pneumonia.

Indications. In tuberculosis, as noted, some feel expectorated sputum is a better diagnostic specimen source in patients with a productive cough. Nevertheless, the yield with bronchoscopy has been reported as high as 32 of 34 (94%) and for atypical mycobacteria the yield was 38 of 40 (96%) (41,47,64).

The diagnostic yield for *P. carinii* is 95% in patients with AIDS and somewhat lower in other patient populations (46,65).

The major setting for cytomegalovirus (CMV) is pneumonitis in a marrow or organ transplant recipient (66).

In the immunocompromised host, the yield according to aggregate data from multiple studies from over 1200 patients showed a diagnostic yield of 30%–55% and false-negative cultures in 21%–35% (41).

For nosocomial pneumonia, bronchoscopy specimens obtained by the protected brush catheter or BAL using quantitative cultures is now being used with increasing frequency to define the presence and cause of bacterial infection, especially in the ICU and in intubated patients. Particularly interesting is a report using this technique to establish the diagnosis suggests that only about 30% of patients with common clinical and radiographic evidence of nosocomial pneumonia actually have supporting evidence based on quantitative culture techniques (67). Major questions in patients receiving mechanical ventilation are the need for bronchoscopy versus suction aspiration, the importance of quantitative verses semiquantitative cultures, and the merit of various stain procedures (68,69).

Chronic or enigmatic pneumonia in the immunocompetent host is also an indication for bronchoscopy.

Community-Acquired Penumonia

Snapshot Summary

Clinical features: Cough, fever and sputum production ± pleurisy.

Diagnosis: New infiltrate on chest radiograph and symptoms of infection.

Diagnostic evaluation

Outpatients: Chest radiograph ± air-dried slide for subsequent stain. Sputum culture is optional.

Candidates for admission: Chest radiograph, air-dried slide for subsequent stain, pulse oximetry or blood gases, chemistry panel.

Hospitalized patients: Chest radiograph, expectorated sputum for Gram stain and culture; blood cultures ×2; AFB stain and culture with cough longer than 1 month and less than 1 year; *Legionella* test (culture, sputum DFA, urinary antigen) if seriously ill, especially if endemic or epidemic or compromised host; complete blood count; chemistry panel including renal and liver function tests and electrolytes; arterial blood gases.

Microbial diagnosis (hospitalized patients)

Blood cultures ×2 prior to antibiotic treatment.

Expectorated sputum—preferably physician procured, deep cough, pretreatment. Specimen should be Gram stained and cultured with incubation within 2–5 hours of collection.

Legionella: Preferred tests are culture (technically difficult) and urinary antigen (detects *L. pneumophila* serogroup 1 which accounts for 70% of cases; technically easy and remains positive after treatment.

Mycoplasma pneumoniae: Cold agglutinins positive at ≥1:64 in 65% of cases, higher with severe disease; relatively nonspecific.

Chlamydia pneumoniae: No realistic test offered by most laboratories.

Treatment

Antibiotic treatment should be initiated within 2–4 hours of initial evaluation with acute symptoms.

Pathogen directed: See Table 1.9.

Empiric treatment (preferred regimens).

Outpatients: Macrolide (erythromycin, azithromycin, or clarithromycin) or fluoroquinolone (levofloxacin, ofloxacin, or sparfloxacin).

Hospitalized patients: Cefotaxime or ceftriaxone or ampicillin-sulbactam ± macrolide.

Alternative: Fluoroquinolone or clindamycin

ICU admission: Macrolide (erythromycin, azithromycin, or clarithromycin) or fluoroquinolone (levofloxacin, ofloxacin, or sparfloxacin) *plus* cefotaxime, ceftriaxone or a betalactam-betalactamase inhibitor.

Response

The overall mortality rate for patients hospitalized with pneumonia is 10%–12%.

Poor prognostic findings: Advanced age, multiple lobe involvement, leukopenia or leukamoid reaction, alcoholism, bacteremia.

Expected response: Clinical response (subjective) within 2–3 days, afebrile in 3–5 days, negative blood cultures within 48 hours, radiographic clearing in mean of 3–12 weeks depending on host and pathogen.

Prevention: Pneumovax and influenza vaccine with highest priority for persons aged older than 65 years, residents of nursing homes, and persons with cardiopulmonary disease.

INCIDENCE

Surveys of pneumonia in the United States indicate an annual attack rate of approximately 12–15/1000 adults. Of the 4,000,000 per year with a diagnosis of pneumonia, approximately 600,000 (15%) require hospitalization (see Table 1.6) (70). The death rate attributed to community-acquired pneumonia (CAP) in the United States is about 10% of hospitalized patients (71). The crude death rate attributed to influenza and pneumonia in the United States for 1994 was 31.8 deaths per 100,000 population; this represents a 59% increase compared with 20.0 deaths per

Table 1.6 Impact of Community-Acquired Pneumonia in the United States	
Number cases/year	4,000,000
Number patients requiring hospitalization	600,000
Number who die with pneumonia as major cause	75,000
Aggregate cost	$4.4 billion

^aFrom: multiple sources. See references (70) and (71).

100,000 recorded in 1979 (72) (Fig. 1.1). There is no readily apparent explanation for this increase.

DIAGNOSIS

Nearly all patients have fever, symptoms suggesting a lower respiratory tract infection, and a chest radiograph showing an infiltrate. The symptoms of bronchitis or sinusitis with postnasal drainage may be identical, and the only way to distinguish them is with a chest radiograph. The radiograph is important in management decisions because the absence of an infiltrate usually indicates bronchitis, which generally does not require antibiotic treatment; by contrast, virtually all forms of pneumonia are treated with antimicrobial

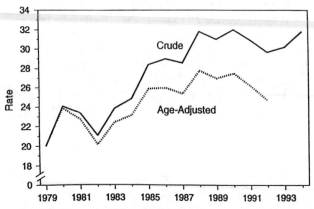

Figure 1.1 Crude and age-adjusted rates of pneumonia and influenza deaths as underlying cause of death in the United States from 1979 to 1994. Results are based on codes 480-487 of the International Classification of Diseases, Ninth Revision, using codes 480-487. Rates are provided /100,000 population. The rate of 31.8/100,000 in 1993 is significantly higher than the rate of 20/100,000 in 1979. Persons aged 65 years or older accounted for 89% of deaths in 1994 (reference 72).

Table 1.7
Indications for Hospitalization[a]

Severe vital sign abnormality
  Pulse >140/min, systolic blood pressure <90 mm Hg,
    respiratory rate >30/min (46%)[b]
Altered mental status (newly diagnosed)
  Disorientation to person, place or time, stupor or coma
    (20%)
Arterial hypoxemia
  pO_2 <60 mm Hg on room air (51%)
Suppurative pneumonia-related infection
  Empyema, septic arthritis, meningitis, endocarditis (1%)
Severe electrolyte, hematologic, or metabolic laboratory
  value not known to be chronic
  Serum Na^{++} <130 mEq/L, hematocrit <30%, absolute
    neutrophil count <1,000/mm^3, blood urea nitrogen
    >50 mg/dL, or creatinine >2.5 mg/dL (13%)
Acute coexistent medical condition requiring admission (23%)

---

[a]Adapted from: Fine MJ, Arloff JJ, Arisumi D et al: Prognosis of patients hospitalized with community-acquired pneumonia. Am J Med 1990;88:1 and Fine MJ, Auble TE, Yealy DM et al: Prediction rule to identify low risk patients with community-acquired pneumonia. New Engl J Med 1997;336:243.
[b]Indicates the percent of patients hospitalized for community-acquired pneumonia with this observation (Fine MJ et al: Hospitalization decision in patients with community-acquired pneumonia: a prospective cohort study. Am J Med 1990;89:713 (73).

agents. "Walking pneumonia" is a term commonly used in reference to patients who are ambulatory and, by inference, are not very sick. Elderly patients may appear deceptively well despite serious disease as indicated by chest radiograph, bacteremia, or subsequent disease course.

Diagnostic studies advocated for patients who are more seriously ill and considered candidates for hospitalization are summarized in Table 1.2. Indications for hospitalization are summarized in Table 1.7. Such indications repre-

sent a tabulation of signs, symptoms, and laboratory findings that indicate serious, often life-threatening disease.
The percentages given in the table indicate the frequency
that these findings applied to admissions to Massachusetts
General Hospital in a retrospective review of CAP (73).
The validity of these observations for predicting mortality
has been established with a review of 38,039 adults hospitalized with pneumonia in 1991 (70). A conclusion from
this assessment is that 26%–31% of these patients could
have been managed as outpatients. Nevertheless, many patients may require hospitalization who do not necessarily
satisfy these criteria owing to concern for the home support mechanism and the probability of compliance with
management recommendations and follow-up.

MICROBIOLOGY

Major pathogens found in community-acquired pneumonia
are summarized in Table 1.8. These results are based on estimates from the British Thoracic Society (88), a review of
15 published papers on CAP (9,19,74–87), and a meta-
analysis of 122 published papers in the English language
literature from 1966 to 1995 (71). The difference with the
latter two series is that data in 15 of the published reports
are for all patients with ranges for the major pathogens; the
summary of 122 reports represents a meta-analysis in
which results are restricted to the 7,079 who had a likely
causative agent detected. It should be noted that there is a
substantive bias in published reports because most are
based on studies of patients who are sufficiently ill to require hospitalization. In addition, there is substantial variation in the attempts to recover other agents, especially the
atypical agents such as *Legionella* sp., *C. pneumoniae,* and
M. pneumoniae; these organisms are presumably under represented. Of particular interest is the observation that even
with extensive diagnostic studies, nearly all of these reports
show that no likely etiologic diagnosis is established in

Table 1.8
Microbiology of Community-Acquired Pneumonia

Microbial agent	Literature review[a] (%)	British Thoracic Society[b] (%)	Meta-analysis[c] (%)
Bacteria			
Streptococcus pneumoniae	20–60	60–75	65
Haemophilus influenzae	3–10	4–5	12
Staphylococcus aureus	3–5	1–5	2
Gram-negative bacilli	3–10	rare	1
Miscellaneous agents[d]	3–5	(not included)	3
Atypical agents	10–20	—	12
Legionella sp.	2–8	2–5	4
Mycoplasma pneumoniae	1–6	5–18	7
Chlamydia pneumoniae	4–6	(not included)	1
Viral	2–15	8–16	3
Aspiration pneumonia	6–10	(not included)	—
No diagnosis	30–60	—	—

[a]Based on 15 published reports from North America (ref 9, 19, 74–87). Low and high values are deleted for each pathogen.
[b]Estimates based on analysis of 453 adults in prospective study of community-acquired pneumonia in 25 British hospitals (88).
[c]Meta-analysis of 122 reports in the English language literature, 1966–1995; analysis restricted to 7113 cases in which a suspected pathogen was reported (71).
[d]Includes *Moraxella catarrhalis,* group A streptococcus, *Neisseria meningitidis, Coxiella burnetti,* and *Chlamydia psittaci.*

30%–50% of cases. This low yield is ascribed to problems, such as 20%–30% of patients do not provide sputum samples, 20%–30% of patients have received prior antimicrobial agents, some pathogens require specialized techniques for cultivation, and microbiologic methods are often substandard as has been discussed (82).

The historical perspective on these results is of particular interest. In the prepenicillin era, *S. pneumoniae* accounted for about 80% of pneumonia cases (90,91). Many studies reported during the past decade indicate a yield of only 10%–20% for *S. pneumoniae* (9,82–87), suggesting that this organism is either disappearing, other agents are taking over, or laboratory techniques for its recovery are now relatively poor. The truth is probably some combination of these observations, but compelling data suggest that pneumococcus is far more important than the more recent experience suggests for the following reasons:

- *S. pneumoniae* still represents the single most commonly defined pathogen in nearly all studies of hospitalized patients with CAP. The meta-analysis of 7079 reported cases in patients who had a causative agent defined showed pneumococcus accounted for 4432 (65%) (71).
- Studies using more aggressive methods to obtain uncontaminated specimens, such as transtracheal aspiration, show much higher yields (31,34,35).
- Studies using more aggressive laboratory methods than are customary to process expectorated sputum also show much higher yields; these include mouse inoculation, plating of specimens on the ward, special care in specimen procurement, and assays of urine, blood, and respiratory secretions for pneumococcal polysaccharide antigen.
- Multiple studies show that the frequency of recovery of *S. pneumoniae* from sputum in patients with bacteremic pneumococcal pneumonia is only about 50% (13–15);

this suggests that the yield in most studies based on expectorated sputum should be at least doubled.

- An analysis by the British Thoracic Society Pneumonia Research Committee concluded after a statistical analysis of 148 patients with no identifiable pathogens that most of these cases were probably due to *S. pneumoniae* (93).

These data suggest that *S. pneumoniae* is far more common than generally reported.

Other commonly encountered bacteria that can be detected with conventional cultures of expectorated sputum are *H. influenzae*, *S. aureus*, and Gram-negative bacilli. Each of these accounts for 3%–10% of cases and each plays a somewhat disputed role owing to the uncertainty of these microbes as pathogens when recovered in expectorated sputum samples.

Less common pathogens are *Moraxella catarrhalis*, *Streptococcus pyogenes*, *Chlamydia psittaci*, *Coxiella burnetti*, and *Neisseria meningitidis*. These organisms usually account for 1%–2% of cases in most series.

Anaerobic bacteria are the dominant pathogens in aspiration pneumonia, lung abscess, and empyema, but they play a very poorly defined role in uncomplicated pneumonia (31,36,37). Our studies using transtracheal aspiration indicate that pneumonitis due to anaerobes could not be easily distinguished from other common forms of bacterial pneumonia based on clinical observations (94). Of particular importance is the observation that two of the relatively important clues to anaerobic infection are not present: tissue necrosis with abscess formation and the presence of putrid discharge. These are common features with late complications, but are not found in early-stage disease and do not evolve if there is adequate management at initial presentation (37). Specifically, analysis of 47 patients with transtracheal aspirations that yielded an exclusive flora of anaerobic bacteria compared with 47 cases yielding only *S. pneumoniae* showed the former group had a more subtle evolution of disease, no reports of shaking chills, and most had associated conditions that predisposed to aspiration. The frequency of anaerobic infections in unselected patients with CAP has been studied using transtracheal aspiration by Reis, et al. showing anaerobes in 29 of 89 patients (33%) (95). A similar yield (38 of 172 patients [22%]) was found by Pollock using quantitative cultures of fiberoptic bronchoscopy aspirates (96). The implication of these observations is that anaerobic bacteria probably account for a significant number of enigmatic pneumonias; furthermore, the diagnostic tests now in common use will never detect anaerobes because upper airway secretion contamination makes the usual specimen sources invalid for meaningful anaerobic culture.

Atypical organisms include *Legionella*, *M. pneumoniae*, and *C. pneumoniae*. The term "atypical pneumonia" was originally used in 1938 by Relman in reference to the organism that was subsequently implicated in "cold agglutinin" pneumonia in the 1940s and then "Eaton agent" pneumonia in the 1950s (97–99). All of these ("atypical pneumonia," "cold agglutinin pneumonia," and "Eaton agent pneumonia") subsequently were shown to be synonymous with *M. pneumoniae* (100,101). More recently, it has become common practice to include *Legionella* and *C. pneumoniae* as "atypical agents." These three organisms collectively account for 10%–20% of all cases, but they show great variation in frequency based on epidemiologic patterns that are temporal and geographic. As will be discussed, the diagnostic techniques to detect atypical agents are evolving. Techniques are available for detection of *Legionella* and all are reasonably specific, but lack sensitivity (102–104). This means that detection by culture, DFA stain, or by urinary antigen assay is adequate for a presumptive diagnosis on which to base therapeutic decisions; the failure to detect *Legionella* by any or all of these techniques is still clearly compatible with this diagnosis (101). *M. pneumoniae* has been found in 1%–8% of patients with CAP who require hospitalization; the rates are much higher for young adults with "walking pneumonia" and there is some suggestion that *Mycoplasma* may be important in elderly patients who require hospitalization. The problem is that most laboratories do not offer diagnostic tests that provide useful information at the time therapeutic decisions are necessary. The same applies to a large extent for *C. pneumoniae* (104–106). This organism reportedly accounts for 5%–10% of cases of CAP, but diagnostic tests are problematic and virtually no clinical laboratories offer these tests.

Viral agents are detected in 2%–15% of cases, most frequently influenza; less commonly, parainfluenza, RSV, and adenovirus. It is expected that viral infections account for a substantial number of pneumonia cases in young, otherwise healthy adults. The problem is the paucity of studies using appropriate diagnostic techniques in this patient population and doubts regarding the sensitivity of current techniques for detecting viral agents that may be fastidious or unknown. In influenza epidemics the yield is obviously much higher. Pneumonia may represent direct viral invasion of the lung (primary influenza pneumonia) or pneumonia may result from secondary bacterial infection, most commonly due to *S. pneumoniae* or *S. aureus* (107,108). Adenovirus types 3 and 21 account for sporadic cases of pneumonia in adults. Parainfluenza virus types 1 and 3 may cause pneumonia in adults, especially in nursing home outbreaks (109–111). RSV is generally considered a pediatric viral infection, but elderly and immunocompromised patients are vulnerable to it (111–113).

THERAPY

Decisions regarding the selection of antibiotics for patients with community-acquired pneumonia is obviously simplified if a microbial diagnosis is established (Table 1.9). The

Table 1.9
Treatment of Pneumonia by Pathogen

Agent	Preferred Antimicrobial	Alternative Antimicrobial Agents
Streptococcus pneumoniae Penicillin-sensitive (MIC <0.1 µg/mL)	Penicillin G or V Amoxicillin	Cephalosporins: Cefazolin, Cefuroxime, Cefotaxime, Ceftriaxone Oral cephalosporins: Cefpodoxime, Cefprozil, Cefuroxime Macrolides[a] Vancomycin Clindamycin Doxycycline
Penicillin-intermediate resistance (MIC 0.1–1 µg/mL)	Penicillin G, 2–3 mIU IV q4h Ceftriaxone, cefotaxime **Oral agents:** Macrolide[a] Fluoroquinolone[a] Clindamycin	Vancomycin Other agents, based on in vitro sensitivity tests

[a]Macrolides: erythromycin, clarithromycin, azithromycin, dirithromycin; Fluoroquinolones: ofloxacin, levofloxacin, sparfloxacin; Betalactam-betalactamase inhibitors: amoxicillin-clavulanic acid, ampicillin-sulbactam, ticarcillin-clavulanic acid, piperacillin-tazobactam
MIC, minimal inhibitory concentration; CMV, cytomeglovirus.

(continued)

Table 1.9 (*continued*)

Agent	Preferred Antimicrobial	Alternative Antimicrobial Agents
Penicillin-high level resistance (MIC >1 μg/mL)	Vancomycin Fluoroquinolone[a]	Imipenem Ceftriaxone Cefotaxime Other agents, based on in vitro sensitivity tests
Empiric selection High risk for penicillin resistance	Vancomycin, Fluoroquinolone[a]	Cephalosporin: Ceftriaxone, Cefotaxime, Cefpodoxime, Cefprozil, Cefuroxime Macrolide Clindamycin Vancomycin Doxycycline
Low risk for penicillin resistance	Penicillin, amoxicillin, cephalosporin, macrolide Fluoroquinolone	
Hemophilus influenzae	Cephalosporin—2nd or 3rd generation TMP-SMX	Betalactam-betalactamase inhibitor[a] Tetracycline Fluroquinolone[a] Azithromycin
Moraxella catarrhalis	Cephalosporin—2nd or 3rd generation TMP-SMX Amoxicillin-clavulanate	Macrolide[a] Fluoroquinolone[a]

(continued)

Table 1.9 *(continued)*

Agent	Preferred Antimicrobial	Alternative Antimicrobial Agents
Anaerobes	Clindamycin Penicillin + metronidazole Betalactam-betalactamase inhibitor	Penicillin G or V Ampicillin/amoxicillin Imipenem/meropenem
Staphylococcus aureus Methicillin-sensitive	Nafcillin/oxacillin ± rifampin or gentamycin	Cefazolin or cefuroxime Vancomycin, clindamycin, TMP-SMX, Fluoroquinolone[a] (if sensitive in vitro)
Methicillin-resistant	Vancomycin ± rifampin or gentamycin	Requires in vitro testing: Fluoroquinolones, TMP-SMX
Enterobacteriaceae[b] (Coliforms: Escherichia coli; Klebsiella, Proteus, Enterobacter, etc.)	Cephalosporin—2nd or 3rd generation ± amino- glycoside	Aztreonam, imipenem, betalactam- betalactamase inhibitor antipseudomonal penicillin (ticarcillin, piperacillin) Fluoroquinolone
Pseudomonas aeruginosa[b]	Aminoglycoside + antipseu- domonal betalactam: Ticarcillin, piperacillin, mezlocillin, ceftazidine	Aminoglycoside + aztreonam, imipenem, or fluoroquinolone
Legionella	Erythromycin ± rifampin	Clarithromycin or azithromycin + rifampin Doxycycline + rifampin
	Fluoroquinolone[a]	

[b]In vitro sensitivity tests needed for optimal treatment.

(continued)

Table 1.9 *(continued)*

Agent	Preferred Antimicrobial	Alternative Antimicrobial Agents
Mycoplasma pneumoniae	Doxycycline Erythromycin	Clarithromycin or azithromycin Fluoroquinolone[a]
Chlamydia pneumoniae	Doxycycline Erythromycin	Clarithromycin or azithromycin Fluoroquinolone[a]
Chlamydia psittaci	Doxycycline	Chloramphenicol
Nocardia	Sulfonamide TMP-SMX	Sulfonamide + minocycline or amikacin Imipenem ± amikacin Doxycycline or minocycline
Coxiella burnetti (Q fever)	Tetracycline	Chloramphenicol
Influenza A	Amantadine or Rimantadine	
Hantavirus	Supportive care (inotropics and vasopressors)	Ribavirin (experimental)
Cytomegalovirus	Ganciclovir ± IVIG or CMV hyperimmune globulin	Foscarnet ± IVIG or CMV hyperimmune globulin
Pneumocystis carinii	TMP-SMX	Dapsone + trimethoprim Clindamycin + primaquin Atovaquone Pentamidine

optimal tests are those that provide immediately available information to guide the initial decision regarding therapy. Specimen sources in this category include Gram stains, Quellung stain, AFB stain, DFA stains, other antigen detection methods, and polymerase chain reaction (PCR). The usual algorithm for hospitalized patients with CAP is presented in Figure 1.2. Conventional bacterial cultures usually require 24–48 hours and may be particularly important for detecting organisms that require in vitro sensitivity testing. Blood cultures are indicated in patients who are seriously ill, and the yield in most reports for hospitalized patients is 5%–15% (9,19,74–87) with an average of 11% (71). This information usually becomes available at 12–24 hours. Gram stain of pleural fluid provides immediate information in patients with empyema, but less than 1% of patients have this complication. Serologic tests requiring acute and convalescent sera are generally useless in terms of therapeutic decisions. A possible exception is IgM

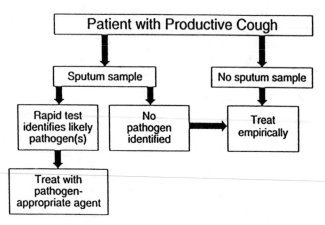

Figure 1. 2 Algorithm for evaluation of pneumonia in hospitalized patients.

for *M. pneumoniae;* cold agglutinin assays may also provide useful information that is immediately available if the titer is 1:64 or greater and the clinical features are supportive.

Guidelines for empiric treatment of pneumonia have been provided by the American Thoracic Society (ATS) (1) and the British Thoracic Society (BTS) (2) as summarized in Table 1.10; the author's recommendations are summarized in Table 1.11. Dose recommendations for suggested agents are listed in Table 1.12. It is curious to note that guidelines from the ATS and BTS are based on analyses of similar published data; both were published in 1993 and both reflect the consensus opinion of authorities in the field. Despite these similarities, the recommendations are quite different.

The guidelines of the British Thoracic Society emphasize the paramount position of *S. pneumoniae* as the most common causative agent and the most common cause of life-threatening pneumonia. This document endorses penicillin and amoxicillin as preferred agents in most patients because such was appropriate for suspected or established pneumococcal pneumonia in England in 1993. The subsequent experience with *S. pneumoniae* shows escalating resistance to penicillin as well as other antimicrobial agents (Table 1.13) (114–119). The recommendations of the American Thoracic Society are based on the severity of illness, age, and associated conditions. The preferred drug for outpatients aged less than 60 years with no comorbidity is erythromycin for its activity against *Mycoplasma, C. pneumoniae,* and *S. pneumoniae;* alternatives include clarithromycin or azithromycin owing to better gastrointestinal tolerance and for some patients who have possible infections with *H. influenzae.* Outpatients aged more than 60 years or who have comorbidity should receive a second generation cephalosporin, trimethoprim-sulfamethoxazole, or a betalactam-betalactamase inhibitor. These drugs are directed against

Table 1.10
Recommendations for Empiric Treatment
of Community-Acquired Pneumonia

The British Thoracic Society (1993) (2)

1. Uncomplicated pneumonia of unknown cause without features indicating severe or nonpneumococcal disease.
   Preferred: an aminopenicillin: amoxicillin, 500 mg PO TID or ampicillin, 500 mg IV QID *or* benzylpenicillin, 1.2 g IV QID.
   Alternatives: Erythromycin, 500 mg PO or IV QID or 2nd or 3rd generation cephalosporin (cefuroxime or cefotaxime).
2. Severe pneumonia of unknown etiology.
   Preferred: erythromycin 1 g IV qid plus 2nd or 3rd generation cephalosporin (cefuroxime, 1.5 g or cefotaxime, 2 g IV TID).
   Alternative: Ampicillin 1 g, flucloxacillin 2 g, and erythromycin 1 g, all IV QID.

American Thoracic Society (1993) (1)

1. Outpatient pneumonia without comorbidity* and age ≤60 years.
   Preferred: Macrolide—erythromycin; alternative (clarithromycin or azithromycin) with erythromycin intolerance and smokers (to treat *Hemophilus influenzae*)
   Alternative: tetracycline.
2. Outpatient pneumonia with comorbidity[a] and/or age ≥60 years.
   Second generation cephalosporin, trimethoprimsulfamethoxazole, *or* betalactam-betalactamase inhibitor ± erythromycin or other macrolide if *Legionella* suspected.
3. Hospitalized patients.
   Second or 3rd generation cephalosporin *or* betalactambetalactamase inhibitor ± erythromycin if Legionellosis is a concern; rifampin may be added if *Legionella* is documented.
4. Severe community-acquired pneumonia.
   Macrolide (with rifampin if Legionellosis) *plus* 3rd generation antipseudomonad cephalosporin or other antipseudomonad therapy including imipenem or ciprofloxacin *plus* aminoglycoside (≥3 d).

Table 1.11
Empiric Antibiotic Selection

Outpatient

> *Preferred:* macrolide[a] or fluoroquinolone[b] or doxycycline
> *Alternative options:* Amoxicillin-clavulanate, or selected
> 2nd generation cephalosporins (cefuroxime, cefpo-
> doxime, cefprozil)

Hospitalized Patient

Patients treated on hospital ward
> *Preferred:* cefotaxime ± macrolide *or* ceftriaxone ±
> macrolide *or* ampicillin-sulbactam ± macrolide
> *Alternatives:* fluoroquinolone[b] or clindamycin (if aspira-
> tion suspected)

Hospitalized patients in intensive care unit for serious pneumonia
> *Preferred:* macrolide[a] or fluoroquinolone[b]
> PLUS
> cefotaxime *or*
> ceftriaxone *or*
> betalactam-betalactamase inhibitor
> *Alternatives:* vancomycin (if high rates of resistance to ce-
> fotaxime and ceftriaxone in community) *or* fluoro-
> quinolone[b] ± clindamycin (penicillin allergy)

[a]Macrolide: erythromycin, clarithromycin, or azithromycin;
azithromycin is preferred when *Hemophilus influenzae* is suspected.
[b]Fluoroquinolone: ofloxacin, levofloxacin, or sparfloxacin.

common bacterial agents, but lack activity against atypical agents. There is the option to add erythromycin if
Legionella is suspected.

Both the ATS and the BTS recommend macrolide therapy for patients who have severe and life-threatening CAP
based on the concern for *Legionella* as an important cause
of life-threatening infection. Additional agents are combined with the macrolide to cover common bacterial
pathogens. The ATS guidelines include treatment directed

Table 1.12
Dose Regimens of Commonly Used Antimicrobials for Community-Acquired Pneumonia

Agent	Usual adult dose	
	Oral	Parenteral
MACROLIDES		
Erythromycin	250–500 mg QID	1 g IV q6h
Clarithromycin (Biaxin)	250–500 mg BID	—
Azithromycin (Zithromax)	500 mg, then 250 mg QD ×4	—
Dirithromycin		
PENICILLINS		
Penicillin V	500 mg QID	—
Penicillin G	500 mg QID	500,000–2 mU q4–6h
Ampicillin	500 mg QID	1–2 g IV q6h
Amoxicillin	250–500 mg TID	—
Oxacillin/nafcillin	500 mg QID	1–3 g IV q6h
Ticarcillin (Ticar)	—	3–6 g IV q6h
Piperacillin (Pipracil)	—	3–6 g IV q6h
Mezlocillin (Mezlin)	—	3–6 g IV q6h
CEPHALOSPORINS		
1st generation		
Cefazolin	—	0.75–2 g IV or IM q8h
Cephalexin (Suprex)	250–500 mg QID	—
Cephradine	250–500 mg QID	1–2 g IV q6h
2nd generation		
Cefuroxime (Ceftin)	250–500 mg BID	750–1500 mg IV q8h
Cefaclor (Ceclor)	250–500 mg TID	—

(continued)

Table 1.12 *(continued)*

| Agent | Usual adult dose | |
	Oral	Parenteral
3rd generation		
Cefotaxime (Claforan)	—	1–3 g q6h
Ceftizoxime (Cefizox)	—	1–3 g q6h
Ceftriaxone	—	500 mg–1 g q12–24 hrs
Ceftazidime	—	1–2 g/day
Cefixime (Suprex)	400 mg QD	—
Cefprozil (Cefzil)	500 mg QD or BID	—
Cefpodoxime (Vantin)	100–400 mg BID	—
4th generation		
Miscellaneous beta-lactams		
Imipenem	—	0.5–1 g q6h
Loracarbef (Lorabid)	200–400 mg BID	—
BETALACTAM-BETALACTAMASE INHIBITORS		
Amoxicillin-clavulanate (Augmentin)	0.25–0.75 mg q8h of 0.875 mg bid	—
Ampicillin-sulbactam (Unasyn)	—	1–2 g IV q6h
Ticarcillin-clavulanate (Ticar)	—	3–6 g q h
AMINOGLYCOSIDES		
Gentamicin (Garamycin)	—	1.7 mg/kg q8h or 5–6 mg/kg/day

(continued)

Table 1.12 *(continued)*

Agent	Usual adult dose	
	Oral	Parenteral
AMINOGLYCOSIDES *(continued)*		
Tobramycin (Nebcin)	—	1.7 mg/kg q8h or 5–6 mg/ kg/day
Amikacin (Amikin)	—	5.0 mg/kg q8h or 20 mg/kg/d
FLUORO- QUINOLONES		
Levofloxacin	500 mg qd	500 mg IV q24h
Sparfloxacin	200–400 mg q12h	—
Ciprofloxacin (Cipro)	500–750 mg q12h	200–400 mg IV q12h
Ofloxacin (Floxin)	400 mg q12h	300–400 mg IV q12h
MISCELLANEOUS		
Trimethoprim- sulfamethoxazole	1 DS BID	2–20 mg/kg (TMP) q6h
Doxycycline (Vibramycin)	100 mg BID	100 mg IV BID
Rifampin	300 mg BID	600 mg IV qd
Metronidazole (Flagyl)	250–500 mg q12h	250–500 IV q 6–12 hrs
Vancomycin	—	1 g IV q12h

against *Pseudomonas aeruginosa* for patients who are seriously ill, although *P. aeruginosa* would be an extraordinarily rare pathogen in this setting except in patients with bronchiectasis, cystic fibrosis, advanced HIV infection, or

Table 1.13
Streptococcus pneumoniae

In Vitro Susceptibility Based on Analysis of 1537 Clinically Significant
Strains from 30 Participating Centers in the U.S. 1994–95 (114)

Agent	Resistant (%)
Penicillin	24
Intermediate	14
High level	10
Cephalosporins[a]	
Cefotaxime	3
Ceftriaxone	5
Cefuroxime	12
Trimethoprim-sulfamethoxazole	18
Tetracycline	8
Chloramphenicol	4
Vancomycin	0

In Vitro Susceptibility Based on Analysis of Isolates from 431 Patients
with Invasive Disease in Metropolitan Atlanta in 1993 (115)

Agent	Resistance (no. resistant among 431 strains tested)	Resistance of penicillin-resistant strains (109 strains)
Penicillin		
Intermediate	77 (18%)	
High level	32 (7%)	
Cefotaxime	37 (9%)	37 (34%)
Cefaclor	61 (14%)	59 (54%)
Erythromycin	66 (15%)	45 (41%)
Trimethoprim-sulfamethoxazole	110 (26%)	82 (75%)
Chloramphenicol	13 (3%)	13 (12%)
Clarithromycin	63 (15%)	
Ofloxacin	4 (1%)	1 (1%)
Tetracycline	34 (8%)	26 (24%)
Imipenem	25 (6%)	25 (23%)

[a]Rank order of activity of cephalosporins beginning with most active
ceftriaxone = cefotaxime ≥ cefpodoxime ≥ cefuroxime >cefprozil
≥ cefixime > cefaclor = loracerbef > cefadroxil = cephalexin.

neutropenia. In the meta-analysis of 7079 cases of CAP by Fine, et al. (71), all Gram-negative bacteria combined accounted for only 1% of all cases.

The sharp differences in these two guidelines illustrate nicely the difficulty in achieving consensus agreement for the empiric treatment of community-acquired pneumonia even by authorities in the field. Criticisms of these guidelines have emphasized three points:

1. The ATS guidelines do not recommend microbiologic studies either owing to distrust of the utility of laboratory technology for detecting likely causative agents or because this information is felt to be superfluous. This impression may reflect the current state-of-the-art regarding a microbial diagnosis, although many would interpret this observation as a mandate for improved laboratory standards with better quality assurance rather than reliance on empiric decisions. One of the major problems with empiricism to the exclusion of microbiology is the need for broad spectrum agents, the inherent lack of epidemiologic data on important pathogens, and the inability to verify sensitivity profiles including the important issue of antibiotic resistance by *S. pneumoniae* and, to a lesser extent, *S. aureus*.

2. The ATS and BTS guidelines were written at the dawn of concern for antibiotic resistance by *S. pneumoniae*. As noted, there is compelling evidence that this organism is by far the most common cause of CAP requiring hospitalization. Empiric treatment directed against *S. pneumoniae* is no longer simple owing to widespread resistance to penicillin and many other agents as well (114–117). This observation suggests that these empiric decisions continue to be a moving target that requires adjustment with time and with geographic vagaries in the sensitivity profile of *S. pneumoniae*. Despite this concern, it is admittedly difficult to show that in vitro sensitivity clearly predicts clinical response (119).

3. The specific organisms that have prompted the greatest debate are *S. pneumoniae*, which is the most common pathogen identified in most series and now often resistant to commonly used drugs; *Legionella*, which is rare in patients aged less than 45 years and rare in patients who are not seriously ill enough to require hospitalization; and the advice to direct therapy against *P. aeruginosa* in seriously ill patients. The latter is a point of contention because it is so rare, accounting for less than 0.5% of all cases in the meta-analysis of 122 reports by Fine (71); when present and pathogenic, the host usually has concurrent conditions that predict this complication: structural disease of the lung, neutropenia, cystic fibrosis, or advanced AIDS.

The author's recommendations account for these possible deficiencies and are based on updated information to include newly available antimicrobial agents and sensitivity patterns of penicillin-resistant *S. pneumoniae* (see Tables 1.13,1.14). It should be emphasized that these recommendations are appropriate for empiric treatment; pathogen-directed therapy is preferred when this information is available.

RESPONSE AND OUTCOME

Both the response and outcome of patients with community-acquired pneumonia depend to a large extent on the microbial agent involved and the host status. Poor prognostic factors based on host status, clinical features, and laboratory findings for CAP are summarized in Table 1.15 (2,83, 120,121) and mortality by microbial pathogen is summarized in Table 1.16 (71).

The greatest experience is with pneumococcal pneumonia. Following initiation of penicillin treatment with penicillin-sensitive *S. pneumoniae*, most patients show clinical improvement within 24–48 hours with decrease in temperature and reduction in systemic toxicity (122). The

Table 1.14
Activity of Commonly Advocated Antimicrobial Agents Versus Common Agents of Pneumonia[a]

	Streptococcus pneumoniae	Hemophilus influenzae	Staphylococcus aureus	Anaerobes (AnO2)	Gram-negative bacillus	Mycoplasma pneumoniae	Chlamydia pneumoniae	Legionella
Amoxicillin	++	++	++	++	+	—	—	—
Tetracycline	++	+++	++	++	+	+++	+++	++
Erythromycin	++	+	++	++	—	+++	+++	+++
Azithromycin	++	+++	++	++	—	+++	+++	+++
Cefotaxime	++	+++	+++	+	++	—	—	—
Cefuroxime	++	+++	++	+	++	—	—	—
TMP-SMX	+	+++	+++	—	+	—	—	—
Levofloxacin	+++	+++	+++	—	++	+++	++	++

+ + + = good in vitro activity; + + = moderate activity, active vs. most strains; + = reduced activity; — = poor activity.

Table 1.15
Poor Prognostic Factors for Patients with Pneumonia[a]

Age: >65 years
Coexisting disease
  Diabetes, renal failure, heart failure, chronic lung disease,
  chronic alcoholism, hospitalization within 1 year previously, immunosuppression, neoplastic disease
Clinical findings
  Respiratory rate >30/min
  Systolic pressure <90 mm Hg or diastolic <60 mm Hg
  Fever >38.3°C
  Altered mental status (lethargy, stupor, disorientation, coma)
  Extrapulmonary site of infection: meningitis, septic arthritis, etc.
Laboratory tests
  White blood count <4,000/dL or >30,000/dL
  PaO_2 <60 mm Hg on room air
  Renal failure
  Chest radiograph showing multiple lobe involvement, rapid spread or pleural effusion
  Hematocrit <30%
Microbial pathogens
  Streptococcus pneumoniae
  Legionella

---

[a]Adapted from: American Thoracic Society. Guidelines for the initial management of adults with community-acquired pneumonia: diagnosis, assessment of severity, and initial antimicrobial therapy. Am Rev Respir Dis 1993;148:1418; Fine MJ, Smith DN, Singer DE. Hospitalization decision in patients with community-acquired pneumonia. Am Med 1990;89:713; Farr BM, Sloman AJ, Fisch MJ. Predicting death in patients hospitalized for community-acquired pneumonia. Ann Intern Med 1991;115:428.

mean duration of fever is approximately 5 days. The time to resolution of changes on chest radiograph depends largely on the host (123). Young and previously healthy adults show a mean time to a clear chest radiograph of

Table 1.16
Mortality of Community-Acquired Pneumonia[a]

Etiologic Agent	Cases	Mortality	Total Mortality
Streptococcus pneumoniae	4432	545 (12.3%)	65.1%
Hemophilus influenzae	883	65 (7.4%)	7.8%
Staphlococcus aureus	157	50 (31.8%)	6.0%
Legionella	272	40 (14.7%)	4.8%
Klebsiella	56	20 (35.7%)	2.3%
Psudomonas aeruginosa	18	11 (61.1%)	1.3%
Chlamydia pneumoniae	41	10 (9.8%)	1.1%
Mycoplasma pneumoniae	507	7 (1.4%)	0.8%
Mixed bacterial species	301	71 (23.6%)	8.5%
Miscellaneous bacteria	446	18	2.1%
TOTAL	7113	837 (11.8%)	

[a]Adapted from: Fine MJ, Smith MA, Carson SA, et al. Prognosis and outcomes of patients with community-acquired pneumonia JAMA 1995;274:134. Analysis is restricted to cases in which pathogen was reported. Some pathogens are obviously underreported owing to failure to use microbiological techniques for their detection. This especially applies to *M. pneumoniae, Legionella,* and *C. pneumoniae.*

3 weeks; older patients and those with complicated infections show an average of 12 weeks to radiograph clearing (7,121). There is a subset of pneumococcal pneumonia patients who do poorly. Poor prognostic features include multiple lobe involvement, bacteremia, background of alcoholism, age over 60 years, concomitant disease, and neutropenia or a leukamoid reaction. Since the introduction of

penicillin studies have shown that it has obviously had a notable impact on outcome; nevertheless, there is also good evidence that penicillin and other antibiotics have had little effect on the mortality rate during the first 5 days of treatment in patients with bacteremic pneumococcal pneumonia (124). The overall mortality rate of pneumococcal pneumonia among patients hospitalized with this diagnosis is 12% and for patients with bacteremic pneumococcal pneumonia it is 20%–30% (71).

Patients with mycoplasmal pneumonia usually become afebrile within 1–2 days after treatment with tetracycline or a macrolide. Extrapulmonary signs and symptoms usually respond more slowly and the role of antibiotics for

Table 1.17
Response to Therapy in Hospitalized Patients[a]

Pathogen	Mortality (%)	Average LOS (days)	Time to defervesence (mean)	Mean time to radiograph clearance
Streptococcus pneumoniae	12	5–6	3–5	3–13 wks (see text)
Hemophilus influenzae	7	6	2–4	—
Gram-negative bacilli	35–60	11	—	—
Legionella	15–25	—	5	11 wks
Mycoplasma pneumoniae	1	—	1–2	1–2 wks
Pneumocystis carinii	17	8	6	5–8 wks

[a]Data based on: Fine MJ, Smith MA, Carson CA, et al. Prognosis and outcomes of patients with community-acquired pneumonia. JAMA 1995;274:134; Bartlett JG. IDCP Guidelines lower respiratory tract infections. Infectious Disease Clinic Practice 1996;5:147.

these complications is unclear. The mortality rate is virtually nil, although some patients with sickle cell disease and some elderly patients may have relatively severe disease. *Legionella pneumonia* is like serious pneumococcal pneumonia in the sense that many patients have progressive disease despite appropriate antibiotic therapy. The reported mortality is 15%–25% even with erythromycin treatment (71,102,103).

Patients with persistent fever and progressive symptoms after 3–5 days of treatment must be considered possible therapeutic failures if no causative diagnosis was established. Diagnostic considerations in this clinical setting are summarized in Table 1.18. In many instances, the infection

---

Table 1.18
Causes of Failure to Respond to Treatment

1. Disease is too far advanced at time of treatment or treatment is delayed too long: Most common with pneumonia due to *Streptococcus pneumoniae*, *Legionella*, Gram-negative bacilli.
2. Wrong antibiotic selection: Uncommon.
3. Inadequate dose of antibiotic: Most common with aminoglycosides due to failure to use adequate dose or to monitor serum levels.
4. Wrong diagnosis: Noninfectious disease such as pulmonary embolism with infarction, congestive failure, Wegener granulomatosis sarcoid, atelectasis, chemical pneumonitis.
5. Wrong microbial diagnosis.
6. Inadequate host: Debilitated, severe associated disease, immunosuppressed.
7. Complicated pneumonia with undrained empyema, metastatic site of infection (meningitis) or bronchial obstruction (foreign body, carcinoma).
8. Pulmonary superinfection: Most patients respond and then deteriorate with new fever.

has progressed too far by the time treatment was initiated or else the patient is an inadequate host due to debility, immunosuppression, or associated diseases that preclude clinical response. Nevertheless, a diagnostic evaluation is necessary to exclude alternative treatable conditions.

The diagnostic evaluation of the patient who fails to respond usually consists of sequential cultures of expectorated sputum or some other specimen from the respiratory tract in combination with respiratory support (41,126). Cultures of respiratory secretions from any source (expectorated sputum, bronchoscopic aspirates, transtracheal aspirates, or transthoracic aspirate) are likely to be misleading owing to the inherent problem of post-treatment cultures with false-negative results for fastidious pathogens and false-positive results for contaminants. Most studies show that the yield of Gram-negative bacilli or *S. aureus* is 25%–50% when specimens are collected after common forms of antibiotic treatment (27). This usually represents "sputum superinfection" rather that patient superinfection. Nevertheless, it is often difficult for physicians to resist adding new antibiotics with each new organism that represents a potential pathogen in the lower airways.

Diagnostic studies that may be useful include laboratory tests for selected pathogens, such as *Legionella, Mycobacteria,* pathogenic fungi, or *P. carinii.* Fiberoptic bronchoscopy and other techniques may be used to detect noninfectious conditions, such as bronchogenic neoplasms, atelectasis, chemical pneumonitis, interstitial lung disease, sarcoidosis, and so forth. Additional diagnostic tests to consider are computerized tomography using either contrast or high resolution technology. The goal is to detect pleural effusions, cavitary lung disease, adenopathy, and other anatomic changes that may change the differential diagnosis (125). If pulmonary embolism is a diagnostic consideration, a reasonable next step is a lung scan and/or pulmonary angiography.

Hospital-Acquired Pneumonia

Snapshot **Summary**

Incidence: 0.5%–1% of all hospitalized patients; 15%–20% of patients in intensive care units. (However, some studies based on quantitative bronchoscopy aspirates concluded that most of the patients with cough, fever, and sputum have alternative diagnoses) (127).

Clinical features: Onset of symptoms more than 48–72 hours after admission; cough, fever, purulent respiratory secretions, and new infiltrate on chest radiograph.

Diagnostic evaluation:
  Chest radiograph
  Blood cultures ×2
  Respiratory secretions: Gram stain and culture
  Bronchoscopy: Routine use of quantitative cultures of BAL or protected swab specimens in ICU-associated pneumonia is debated

Microbiology
  Pseudomonas aeruginosa and *Enterobacteriaceae* (*Klebsiella* sp., *Enterobacter, Proteus,* and so forth)
  Staphylococcus aureus
  Less common: Anaerobic bacteria, *S. pneumoniae, H. influenzae*
  Compromised host: cytomegalovirus (CMV), *Aspergillus*
  Nosocomial outbreaks: Acinetobacter, *S. aureus, P. aeruginosa, Serratia, Enterobacter, Legionella, Aspergillus,* influenza, RSV, tuberculosis

Treatment
  Pathogen-directed: Major pathogens (GNB and *S. aureus)* are easily recovered in respiratory secretions including expectorated sputum, endotracheal or tra-

cheostomy aspirates, and nasopharyngeal or bronchoscopic aspirates. In vitro sensitivity of dominant potential pathogens should guide treatment.

Empiric (seriously ill):

 Aminoglycoside or ciprofloxacin plus antipseudomonad betalactam, betalactam-betalactamase
inhibitor, imipenem/meropenem, or aztreonam

 Vancomycin should be added if organisms resembling
S. aureus are seen on Gram stain or if *S. aureus* is
endemic/epidemic

Prevention

Yes	Maybe	No
Semi-upright position	Sulcrafate in place of H2 agonists or antacids	Selective decontamination
Contact precautions for selected transmittable pathogens	Continuous aspiration of subglottic	Topical antibiotics in respiratory tract secretions

Nosocomial pneumonia accounts for only about 15%
of hospital-acquired infections, but it is the most frequent lethal nosocomial infection. The bacteriology is
unique compared with community-acquired infection. In addition, the hospital can be the focus of important epidemics including *Legionella*, tuberculosis,
and aspergillosis as well as common nosocomial
pathogens such as *P. aeruginosa* and *S. aureus*.

CLINICAL PRESENTATION

The usual presentation is a new pulmonary infiltrate on
chest radiograph combined with evidence of infection with
fever, purulent sputum, and/or leukocytosis. Other pro-
cesses that may give the same findings include congestive

heart failure, pulmonary thromboembolism, atelectasis, drug reactions, pulmonary hemorrhage, and acute respiratory distress syndrome (ARDS).

INCIDENCE

Most reports indicate 0.5%–1.0% of all hospital admissions develop nosocomial pneumonia (126). The rates in surgical and medical intensive care units are generally reported at 15%–20%. Among mechanically ventilated patients the rate is reported at 18%–60% (usually about 20%) with a mortality rate of 50%–90% (126). It should be noted that some of these incidence figures are disputed by the data from Fagon, et al. (127), who used quantitative cultures of fiberoptic bronchoscopy aspirates in patients with typical clinical features of nosocomial pneumonia including fever, purulent sputum, and a new infiltrate on chest radiograph. The results suggested that only about 40% of patients with these clinical findings had the diagnosis confirmed with the microbiology studies. There may be doubt regarding the diagnostic accuracy of the bronchoscopy aspirates in this study, but most patients with negative results were not treated with antibiotics and subsequently recovered; for those patients who had progressive disease and died, autopsies confirmed the absence of pneumonia. This is a potentially important observation because it suggests that data on the frequency of nosocomial pneumonia may be inflated and that many of these patients actually have other conditions such as pulmonary infarction as noted above.

PATHOGENESIS

There are several interrelated factors to explain the high rates of pulmonary infections among hospitalized patients.
1. The hospital setting represents the clustering of highly vulnerable patients. This is especially true in intensive care units where many patients have predisposing pul-

monary conditions, often with intubation which obviously compromises the defense mechanisms of the airways.

2. Many patients are predisposed to aspiration as a result of compromised consciousness due to associated medical conditions and anesthesia. Aspiration is promoted by upper airway and gastrointestinal tract intubation and the supine position.

3. The dominant organisms in nosocomial pneumonia are Gram-negative bacteria, which presumably reach the lower airways either by aspiration of gastric contents or by "microaspiration" of upper airway secretions. The presumed explanation is the propensity for colonization of the upper airways by Gram-negative bacteria as a reflection of serious illness (Table 1.19) (128–133). The classic study to examine pathogenesis used throat cultures to detect asymptomatic carriage of Gram-negative bacilli in various populations (128). Healthy persons, psychiatric patients, physicians, and medical students had colonization rates of 2%–3%. The rate in patients who were moderately ill was 30%–40%, and in the intensive care unit it was 60%–70%. These studies were done exclusively in pa-

Table 1.19
Conditions Associated with Pharyngeal Colonization by Gram-Negative Bacilli

Life-threatening illness	Viral upper respiratory infection
Prolonged hospitalization	Alcoholism
Antibiotic exposure	Diabetes
Advanced age	Coma
Severe debility	Pulmonary disease
Intubation	Azotemia
Major surgery	Neutropenia

tients who were not receiving antibiotics so that other factors dictated these colonization rates. Subsequent work has shown that the likelihood of colonization by Gram-negative bacilli in the upper airways seems to correlate directly with the severity of illness and is found most commonly in patients who are severely ill with coma, uremia, and multiple organ failure; it is less frequent in patients who have diabetes, alcoholism, upper respiratory tract infections, and various functional disabilities (Table 1.19). The presumed source of the bacteria in these cases is the patient's own colonic flora (134) and colonization appears to reflect enhanced binding by Gram-negative bacilli to respiratory epithelial cells, which can be demonstrated in vitro (135,136). Thus, the postulated mechanism is colonization of the upper airways in a patient rendered vulnerable by severe disease with microaspiration as the mechanism seeding the lower airways. An alternative possibility is that these organisms are swallowed; they colonize the stomach in the absence of gastric acid and are subsequently aspirated from the gastric source.

MICROBIOLOGY

The microbiology of nosocomial pneumonia according to multiple studies is summarized in Table 1.20 (136–144). Virtually all reports indicate that Gram-negative bacteria account for 50%–70% of cases. The most common bacterium within this category is *P. aeruginosa* followed by a diverse array of *Enterobacteriaceae*. Some cases reflect epidemics, especially within intensive care units. These often involve *Acinetobacter, Serratia, Xanthomonas, Pseudomonas* species, and *Enterobacter*.

Staphylococcus aureus is second to Gram-negative bacteria in most studies and accounts for 10%–20% of all nosocomial pneumonias. *S. epidermiditis* is often found in

Table 1.20
Nosocomial Pneumonia: Microbiology[a]

BACTERIA		80%–90%
Gram-negative bacilli	50%–70%	
Pseudomonas aeruginosa[b]		
Enterobacteraceae[b]		
Staphylococcus aureus[b]	15%–30%	
Anaerobic bacteria	10%–30%	
Hemophilus influenzae	10%–20%	
Streptococcus pneumoniae	10%–20%	
Legionella[b]	4%	
VIRAL		10%–20%
Cytomegalovirus		
Influenza[b]		
Respiratory syncytial virus[b]		
FUNGI		<1%
Aspergillus[b]		

[a]From: References 126, 136–145.
[b]May cause nosocomial epidemics.

respiratory secretions, but it has no established pathogenic potential in the lung and should be ignored.

Anaerobic bacteria may be found in up to 20%–30% of cases, but they are not generally sought using appropriate diagnostic specimen sources (139). When they are found, there is usually the concurrent presence of aerobic Gram-negative bacilli or *S. aureus*, and the role of the anaerobes is unclear.

Miscellaneous organisms that have been found in 5%–10% of cases include *S. pneumoniae*, *H. influenzae*, and *C. pneumoniae*.

Legionella has been responsible for approximately 4% of all nosocomial infections according to a multihospital autopsy study in patients with lethal nosocomial pneumonia. Multiple large outbreaks of legionnaires' disease in hospitals are usually traced to water supplies with distribution via air conditioner cooling systems or shower heads (146–148).

Tuberculosis accounts for a relatively small number of nosocomial infections, but obviously represents a major public health problem (149–151). Multiple hospital epidemics have been described; the source is almost invariably patients with unsuspected pulmonary tuberculosis and some nosocomial epidemics have involved multiply drug-resistant strains (149–151). Patients with HIV infection including health care workers are highly vulnerable.

Aspergillosis may occur in epidemics among patients who are vulnerable, usually those who have suppressed cell-mediated immunity and/or neutropenia (152,153). This infection should be suspected when a patient at risk develops a pleural-based lesion that shows characteristic features on CT scan.

DIAGNOSIS

The diagnosis of hospital-acquired pneumonia is usually suspected in patients with fever, respiratory symptoms, and a new infiltrate on chest radiograph. As noted, studies by Fagon et al. suggest that many patients with these findings have alternative diagnoses (67). For practical reasons, many or most will be treated with antibiotics, in part because of the high mortality rate associated with untreated nosocomial pneumonia.

The frequency of bacteremia is 2%–6%, and Gram-negative bacteria are common isolates, often in association with the "sepsis syndrome." All patients should have blood cultures, preferably before antibiotic treatment. In most cases, the only other diagnostic specimen readily available are respiratory secretions with expectorated sputum, naso-pharyngeal aspirates, aspirates of tracheostomies or endotracheal tubes, or bronchoscopic aspirates. A major debate among authorities in the field concerns the utility of bronchoscopy with quantitative cultures in the routine evaluation of suspected pneumonia in ventilated patients ("ventilator-associated pneumonia") in the ICU (68,69).

The dominant pathogens in nosocomial pneumonia are Gram-negative bacilli and *S. aureus,* which are usually easily recovered by culture of respiratory secretions obtained by expectoration, nasotracheal aspiration, or endotracheal tube aspiration. Gram stain of these secretions will give immediate information. Attention should be paid to semi-quantitative culture results using standard microbiology nomenclature of "heavy," "moderate," or "light" growth. The problems noted previously with *S. pneumoniae* in expectorated sputa does not apply to GNB or *S. aureus* because these are hardy organisms that are easily recovered providing the sample originates in the lower airways. A major justification of respiratory secretion cultures is to determine sensitivity test results of the numerically dominant potential pathogens. The major problem is consequently false-positive rather than false-negative culture results so that caution is necessary in decisions about microbial pathogen. The following organisms should usually be ignored because they have no well-recognized role of pulmonary pathogens: *S. epidermidis,* Gram-positive bacilli other than *Nocardia, Hemophilus* species other than *H. influenzae, Micrococcus, Enterococcus,* and *Candida* sp.

THERAPY

Optimal therapy is based on a defined pathogen using cultures of uncontaminated body fluids (pleural fluid or positive blood cultures), quantitative cultures of bronchoscopy aspirates, or suction aspiration of endotracheal or tracheostomy tubes; less conclusive but usually valid are potential pathogens recovered in respiratory secretions obtained by other means, especially if present in large

Table 1.21
Treatment of Nosocomial Pneumonia[a]

Category: mild, early, and low risk
- Mild or moderately severe
- Early onset (<5 hospital days)
- No high risk factors (see Table 1.22)

Cephalosporin: Cefuroxime, cefotaxime, ceftriaxone

Betalactam-betalactamase inhibitor: ampicillin-sulbactam (Unasyn), ticarcillin-clavulanic acid (Timentin), or piperacillin-tazobactam (Zosyn)

Penicillin allergy: Fluoroquinolone or clindamycin plus azithromycin

Category: severe, late, or high risk
- Severe (see Table 1.7 and 1.22)
- Onset >5th hospital day
- High risk (Table 1.22)

Aminoglycoside (gentamicin, tobramycin, amikacin), or ciprofloxacin plus one of the following:

1. Antipseudomonal betalactam: ceftazidime, cefoperazone, cefepine, piperacillin, ticarcillin, mezlocillin
2. Betalactam-betalactamase inhibitor: ticarcillin-clavulanic acid (Timentin), piperacillin-tazobactam (Zosyn)
3. Imipenem or meropenem
4. Aztreonam

With or without: Vancomycin

[a]From: American Thoracic Society. Hospital-acquired pneumonia in adults: diagnosis, assessment of severity, initial antimicrobial therapy and preventive strategies. A consensus statement. Am Rev Respir Crit Care Med 1995;153:1711.
Modified by author to include new antimicrobials: cefepine, meropenam. See Table 1.12 for dose recommendations.

concentrations and seen on direct Gram stain. See Table 1.9 for guidelines by specific microbe and Table 1.12 for dosing recommendations.

Guidelines for empiric treatment based on recommendations of the American Thoracic Society are summarized in Table 1.21 (145). The authors distinguish likely pathogens in patients who have nosocomial pneumonia early in their hospital course (≤5 days), are not severely ill (Table 1.22), and lack specific risk factors. These patients should usually receive a single agent such as a non-antipseudomonas second or third generation cephalosporin, a betalactam-betalactamase inhibitor, or a fluoroquinolone. Empiric treatment in patients who have late onset nosocomial pneumonia or who are seriously ill should be combination antibiotics with antipseudomonad activity with or without vancomycin. Specific risk factors that would modify these recommendations are:

Table 1.22
Definition of Severe Nosocomial Pneumonia[a]

Transfer to intensive care unit for this pneumonia
Respiratory failure
  Need for mechanical ventilation or requirement for >35%
  O_2 to maintain O_2 saturation >90%
Rapid progression on chest radiograph to show multiple
  lobe involvement or cavitation
Evidence of severe sepsis
  Hypotension (systolic <90 mm Hg or diastolic <60 mm Hg)
  Vasopressors required >4 h
  Oliguria with urinary output <20 mL/h
  Acute renal failure requiring dialysis

[a]Adapted from: American Thoracic Society. Hospital-acquired pneumonia in adults: diagnosis, assessment of severity; initial antimicrobial therapy and preventive strategies. A consensus statement. Am Rev Respir Crit Care Med 1995;153:1711.

Risk	Antibiotics Added
Risk of anaerobic infection (Abdominal surgery, observed aspiration or putrid discharge*)	Clindamycin (in combination) or betalactam-betalactamase inhibitor (alone)
Staphylococcus aureus (Coma, head trauma, recent influenza, diabetes, renal failure, injection drug use)	Vancomycin
Legionella (Corticosteroids, endemic or epidemic*)	Erythromycin or cipro-floxacin* ± rifampin
Pseudomonas aeruginosa (Prolonged ICU stay, steroids (?),* antibiotic exposure, structural lung disease, advanced AIDS,* neutropenia*	Treat as described for severe pneumonia

*Added by author

The major criticism of these guidelines is *a)* the emphasis on empiricism and *b)* possibly erroneous conclusions about bacteriologic patterns. Empiric decisions are often unnecessary because a Gram stain of respiratory secretions usually indicates probable pathogens and cultures usually provide the guide to specific antibiotic decisions. This is especially true of respiratory secretions obtained directly from the lower airways: bronchoscopy, endotracheal tube aspiration, or tracheostomy aspirate. The second concern is that the data supporting the concept that microbial patterns are distinctive for early versus late nosocomial pneumonia are not well established (154).

With regard to specific agents, the two pathogens associated with excessive mortality are *P. aeruginosa* and *Acinetobacter* (155,156). *P. aeruginosa* usually is treated with a combination of antibiotics, usually a betalactam plus an aminoglycoside, ciprofloxacin, imipenem, or another beta-lactam. The need for combined treatment for other bacteria is less clear; some authorities use rifampin in combination with a macrolide or fluoroquinolone for *Legionella* (103). For *S. aureus,* some also add low dose gentamicin (1 mg/kg) every 8 hours or rifampin to the betalactam or vancomycin treatment.

Full doses of antimicrobial should be used to assure maximal activity in an infection associated with a high mortality rate. Virtually all antimicrobial agents used for systemic infections penetrate the lung well. A concern is aminoglycosides due to the relatively close toxic-therapeutic ratio (including blood levels that are often marginal or low using standard doses), concern about penetration of these drugs into respiratory secretions, and activity at the acid pH of the lung (145). For these reasons and for fear of nephrotoxicity, many authorities advocate alternative drugs such as cephalosporins, ciprofloxacin, imipenem, or a betalactam-betalactamase inhibitor. When aminoglycosides are used, it is important to verify that therapeutic blood levels are achieved by monitoring peak serum levels at 1 hour after infusion. The goal with tobramycin or gentamicin is a peak of 5 mcg/mL or greater and for amikacin it is 20 mcg/mL or greater (157). An alternative is once daily administration using 5–6 mg/kg/day for tobramycin and gentamicin and 20 mg/kg/day for amikacin.

Outcome. Nosocomial pneumonia is associated with a relatively high mortality rate, usually 8%–20% for all cases; the mortality rate for nosocomial pneumonia acquired in the ICU is 20%–40% with a mean of 26% (145). The attributable mortality is 30-33% meaning that associated conditions are major contributing factors.

Prevention. The substantial risk of pneumonia in medical and surgical ICUs has prompted aggressive methods to prevent this complication. Recommendations are summarized in Table 1.23.

The most important recommendation based on critical analysis of available data is *a)* the use of the semi-upright position to reduce the risk of aspiration and *b)* handwashing between each patient treated to prevent transmission of pathogens (158). The concern for patient positioning is based on marker studies showing a substantial risk of

---

Table 1.23
Prevention of Nosocomial Pneumonia

STRONGLY RECOMMENDED
  Semi-upright position to reduce risk of aspiration
  Contact precautions with mask for the following respiratory tract pathogens
  Bacteria: *Staphylococcus aureus,* group A streptococci, *Neisseria meningitidis,* pertussis, plague, penicillin-resistant *Streptococcus pneumoniae,* multiply resistant Gram-negative bacilli.
  Bacterialike: *Mycoplasma pneumoniae*
  Mycobacteria: *Mycobacterium tuberculosis*
  Viruses: Viral exanthems (measles, rubella, chicken pox, mumps), influenza, enterovirus
  Fungi: None

ENCOURAGED
  Use of sulcrafate in place of H2 agonists or antacids to preserve "gastric barrier"

EXPERIMENTAL
  Continuous aspiration of subglottic secretions in ventilated patients

NOT RECOMMENDED
  Selective decontamination of gastrointestinal tract
  Topical administration (intratracheal instillations or aerosolized administration) of antimicrobial agents

marker displacement from the stomach to the lower respiratory tract associated with the recumbent position compared with the upright or semi-upright position (158). The assumption is that the pathophysiologic mechanism of most cases of nosocomial pneumonia, especially in ICUs, is aspiration of bacteria from the upper airways or stomach.

The second strong recommendation is for infection control using contact precautions with emphasis on handwashing and a mask when exposed to microbial pathogens that are listed in Table 1.23. This is generally regarded as standard infection control policy in most hospitals, although there may be some nuances that are important. For example, *N. meningitidis* is most readily transmitted when it is in respiratory secretions, although only type Y is generally implicated as a cause of pneumonia. Penicillin resistance by *S. pneumoniae* will often not be known for 48 hours, and this may require isolation precautions of patients likely to have pneumococcal pneumonia in areas where resistance is prevalent. Multiply resistant Gram-negative bacilli are generally defined by resistance to aminoglycosides and beta-lactam drugs; most are susceptible to fluoroquinolones and imipenem. An exception is *X. maltophilia,* which is usually susceptible only to trimethoprim-sulfamethoxazole. Viral exanthems are generally transmitted by the respiratory tract in the absence of pulmonary involvement.

It is common practice in intensive care units to administer prophylaxis to prevent peptic ulceration of the stomach. However, neutralization of gastric acid eliminates the "gastric barrier," the acid defense mechanism that prevents colonization of the stomach by various bacteria including GNB. Thus, sucralfate is advocated as a substitute for commonly used H2 agonists or antacids, and the initial experience with this substitution shows a reduction in the frequency of nosocomial pneumonia (159).

A new procedure is continuous aspiration of subglottic secretions in patients receiving ventilation (160). The experience is limited, but the initial report suggests this is another effective mechanism to prevent aspiration pneumonia.

Selective decontamination has been a popular method to interrupt the cycle of colonization of the colon by Gram-negative bacilli followed by colonization of the pharynx by the same organisms with subsequent aspiration either from the upper airways or the gastric contents. The goal of selective decontamination is to eliminate or reduce GNB (and sometimes *S. aureus* and/or *Candida*) in the gastrointestinal tract by antimicrobial agents that will select for these organisms, but preserve the anaerobic bacterial floras that appear critical for population control in the colon. Drugs commonly used are oral administration of polymyxin, aminoglycosides, trimethoprim-sulfamethoxazole, fluoroquinolones, and aztreonam (161). These regimens sometimes include amphotericin B, but oral or systemic administration of imipenem or cephalosporins may be used. An extensive experience with this technique, including 12 controlled trials and over 4000 participants, shows that these regimens effectively reduce the frequency of pneumonia in ICUs, but there is no substantial impact on mortality rates (162). Major concerns with the technique include *a)* failure to reduce mortality rates, *b)* excessive costs of the regimens, and *c)* the perception of antibiotic abuse with the encouragement of resistance. As a result, most authorities now no longer recommend selective decontamination.

Topical antibiotics have also been tested. The topical application to the lower airways is achieved by installation of drugs through tracheostomies or endotracheal tubes, or by aerosolization. The drugs most commonly used are polymyxin or aminoglycosides, although multiple different agents have been given by this route. The most extensive experience was reported by Feely et al. in Boston using polymyxin in an attempt to prevent nosocomial pneumonia due to *P. aeruginosa*. This study showed a reduction in the frequency of Pseudomonas pneumonia, but there was no impact on mortality rates and there was the associated risk of infection involving resistant strains, primarily *Proteus* infections (163). The result of this experience is that topical antibiotics are not recommended. The exception is in patients with cystic fibrosis where this approach to prophylaxis and therapy has documented merit.

Pneumonia in the Compromised Host Including AIDS

Snapshot   Summary

Frequency: Pneumocystis carinii pneumonia (PCP) is the most common initial AIDS-defining complication and pneumonia (presumably bacterial) is the most common cause of death.

Microbiology

CD4 count greater than 200: *S. pneumoniae, S. aureus,* (injection drug users), *H. influenzae, M. tuberculosis*

CD4 count less than 200: Agents above plus *P. carinii, P. aeruginosa, Cryptococcus, Aspergillus, M. kansasii*

Chest radiograph changes: (see Table 1.27)

Clinical presentation

PCP: Subtle onset and progression of dyspnea, fever, and nonproductive cough with CD4 count less than 200/mm³

Pneumococcal pneumonia: Identical to pneumococcal pneumonia in immunocompetent host, but risk is a 100 times greater and rate of bacteremia is higher

Tuberculosis (TB): Typical features with high CD4 count including cough longer than 1 month and less than 1 year, upper lobe infiltrate, ± pleural effusion, adenopathy, and cavity. With CD4 count less than

200/mm^3, there is atypical presentation with lower lobe infiltrates and extrapulmonary disease.

Diagnosis

  Chest radiograph

  CD4 count

  Sputum Gram stain and culture: Acute bacterial pneumonia

  Induced sputum: Primarily for PCP and TB in patients with dry cough

  Bronchoscopy: Optional method to detect PCP

Therapy

  Acute pneumonia with focal infiltrate: Treat as described for community-acquired pneumonia

  PCP established or suspected

    Preferred: Trimethoprim-sulfamethoxazole (TMP-SMX)

    Alternatives: Pentamidine, trimethoprim-dapsone, clindamycin-primaquin, atovaquone

    pO$_2$ less than 70 mm Hg: Prednisone

  TB: Treatment is the same as TB in other populations—four drugs for initial treatment, directly observed treatment preferred, 6-month duration

  Others: See Table 1.26

Prevention

  Pneumovax, preferably with CD4 count greater than 200/mm^3

  PPD positive: oral isoniazide (INH) prophylaxis (lifelong or twelve months)

  PCP prophylaxis: TMP-SMX (preferred; also prevents bacterial pneumonia)

    Alternatives: Dapsone or aerosolized pentamidine

The immunocompromised host now comprises an enlarging component of the patient population. A review of 385 consecutive patients hospitalized at Johns Hopkins Hospital with community-acquired pneumonia in 1991 showed that 216 (56%) were considered immunocompromised (9). Most of these are patients with HIV infection, although 35 of the 180 (19%) were unaware of HIV infection at the time of hospitalization. Given the prevalence and importance of HIV infection, most of this discussion will deal with patients with HIV infection. A summary of microbial pathogens associated with specific host defects is provided in Table 1.24.

INCIDENCE

Pulmonary infections, primarily *P. carinii* pneumonia (PCP), has always been the leading AIDS-defining diagnosis in the United States and it is the most common cause of death found in autopsy series (164). Tuberculosis also represents a major cause of morbidity and mortality, and in many parts of the world this is the most common serious complication of HIV infection. The rates of pneumococcal pneumonia are multiplied at least 100 times in patients with HIV infection compared with the general population. Pneumonia of unknown cause, but presumably bacterial, is now the most common cause of death in patients with HIV infection (164,165). These data indicate the lung is the most common target organ for opportunistic infections in patients with HIV infection.

MICROBIOLOGY

Results of a large multicenter study of pulmonary complications of HIV infection are listed in Table 1.25 (9,46,166). This represents the experience in the United States according to a consensus review in 1985 and an updated review of a second meeting of authorities in 1988. The latter review showed TB was more important than originally thought, and *Legionella* was probably over represented, although more recent experience strongly supports an association based on Centers for Disease Control (CDC) data showing an odds ratio of 41 compared with

Table 1.24
Pulmonary Infections in the Compromised Host: Microbial Associations with Specific Defects

Condition	Usual conditions	Pathogens
Neutropenia (500/mL)	Cancer chemotherapy, adverse drug reaction, leukemia	**Bacteria:** Aerobic GNB (coliforms and pseudomonads), *Staphylococcus aureus*, *Streptococcus viridans*, *Staphylococcus epidermidis* **Fungi:** Aspergillus
Cell-mediated immunity	Organ transplantation, HIV infection; lymphoma (especially), Hodgkin's disease), corticosteroid therapy	**Bacteria:** *Listeria, Salmonella, Nocardia,* Mycobacteria (*M. tuberculosis* and *M. avium*), *Legionella* **Viruses:** CMV, Herpes simplex, Varicella-zoster **Parasites:** *Pneumocystis carinii, Toxoplasma, Strongyloides stercoralis,* Cryptosporidia **Fungi:** Cryptococcus, Histoplasma, Coccoides
Hypogamma-globulinemia or dysgamma-globulinemia	Multiple myeloma, congenital or acquired deficiency, chronic lymphocytic leukemia	**Bacteria:** *Streptococcus pneumoniae, Hemophilus influenza* (type B)

GNB, Gram-negative bacilli; CMV, cytomegalovirus.

(continued)

Table 1.24 (continued)

Condition	Usual conditions	Pathogens
		Bacteria:
Complement deficiencies	Congenital	
C2, 3		*S. pneumoniae, H. influenzae*
C5		*S. pneumoniae, S. aureus, Enterobacteriaceae*
C6–8		*Neisseria meningitidis*
Alternative pathway		*S. pneumoniae, H. influenzae*
Hyposplenism	Splenectomy; hemolytic anemia	*S. pneumoniae, H. influenzae*
Defective chemotaxis	Diabetes, alcoholism, renal failure, lazy leukocyte syndrome, trauma, systemic lupus erythematosus	*S. aureus,* streptococci
Defective neutrophilic killing	Chronic granulomatous disease, myeloperoxidase deficiency	Catalase-positive bacteria: *S. aureus*

Table 1.25
Pulmonary Disorders in Patients with HIV Infection

Pathogen	Multicenter study[a] (441 patients)	Johns Hopkins Hospital[b] (180 patients)
Pneumocystis carinii	373 (85%)	48 (27%)
Cytomegalovirus	74 (17%)	8 (4%)
Myobacterium avium	74 (17%)	—
Kaposi sarcoma	36 (8%)	—
Legionella	19 (4%)	6 (3%)
Myobacterium tuberculosis	19 (4%)	4 (2%)
Fungi	17 (4%)	2 (1%)
Streptococcus pneumoniae	—	38 (21%)
Hemophilus influenzae	—	11 (6%)
Bacteria (other)	—	18 (10%)
No pathogen	—	45 (25%)

[a]Murray JF, Felton CP, Garay SM, et al. Pulmonary complications of the acquired immunodeficiency syndrome. N Engl J Med 1984;310:1682.
[b]Mundy LM, Auwaeter PG, Oldach D, et al. Community-acquired pneumonia: impact of immune status. Am J Respir Crit Care Med 1995;152:1309.

the general population (167). The experience in other countries may be quite different, as noted above. For example, in Africa it appears that TB is the most common pulmonary pathogen and PCP is relatively uncommon (168).

Pneumocystis carinii pneumonia. The experience in the United States suggests that PCP will occur in 70%–80% of all patients with HIV infection in the absence of adequate prophylaxis. PCP has represented the most common initial AIDS-defining diagnosis during every year of the epidemic, although its relative frequency has decreased from about 75% in 1984 to 25% in 1995; the marked decline presumably reflects the widespread use of PCP prophylaxis in patients with HIV infection. Nearly all patients have a CD4 cell count less than 200/mm^3; the average CD4 cell count is approximately 100/mm^3 in patients not receiving prophylaxis and it is about 20/mm^3 in patients receiving recommended prophylaxis. Patients with CD4 counts less than 200/mm^3 should take PCP prophylaxis, preferably with TMP-SMX in a dose of one double strength (DS)/day (169). Alternatives are TMP-SMX in reduced dosage, dapsone (100 mg/day), or aerosolized pentamidine (300 mg/mo). Patients taking PCP prophylaxis have reduced rates of PCP, reduced severity of illness when "breakthroughs" occur, and substantial reductions in health care costs (170).

Pneumococcal pneumonia. The frequency of pneumococcal pneumonia and pneumococcal bacteremia is multiplied at least 100 times in patients with HIV infection (165). This may occur in relatively early stages of disease when the CD4 cell count is 200–400/mm^3, but the frequency of pneumococcal pneumonia increases as immunosuppression increases. The rate is also influenced by the frequent use of prophylactic antibiotics, such as trimethoprim-sulfamethoxazole, azithromycin, and clarithromycin, taken for other conditions in advanced disease (171).

Tuberculosis. Rates of TB are multiplied over 100 times in patients with HIV infection. Studies in the United States indicate high rates of latent TB reactivation; this rate is estimated at 10% per lifetime in patients without HIV infection and nearly 10% per year in those with AIDS (172). Unlike most opportunistic infections, TB is common at relatively high CD4 counts, an average of 200–300/mm^3 in most studies. There is also great vulnerability for progressive primary TB following exposure. Most cases of multiply-drug resistant TB (MDRTB) have involved HIV-infected persons.

Miscellaneous organisms. Other bacterial pathogens in HIV-infected persons with pneumonia include *Nocardia, H. influenzae, S. aureus, Legionella, P. aeruginosa,* and *Rhodococcus equi.* Mycobacteria other than tuberculosis (MOTT) that cause infections in patients with HIV infection include *M. avium, M. kansasii,* and a host of other mycobacteria.

Fungal infections of the lung that are relatively common in AIDS patients include *Cryptococcus, Aspergillus,* and the pathogenic fungi in endemic areas (histoplasmosis, coccidioidomycosis, and blastomycosis).

Viral infections of the lung include CMV, but most of these are cases where the organism is detected, but its role as a pulmonary pathogen is unclear. In addition, it is not clear that these patients respond to standard therapy for CMV infection.

DIAGNOSIS

The differential diagnosis in patients with HIV infection and symptoms of a respiratory tract infection are based on the stage of disease as indicated by the CD4 cell count, the tempo of the lung infection, clinical features of the infection, and changes on chest radiograph.

Characteristic features of various infections are summarized in Table 1.26, based on the tempo of the disease, the epidemiologic setting, the CD4 cell count, and diagnostic tests of choice. In general, patients with PCP report an indolent infection characterized by fever, a nonproductive cough, and progressive dyspnea over a period of weeks prior to medical presentation. Other indolent pulmonary infections include nocardiosis, TB, MOTT, and fungal infections. Acute respiratory tract infections are usually due to bacterial pathogens such as *S. pneumoniae* and, less frequently, *H. influenzae, Legionella,* and *S. aureus. P. aeruginosa* is an important pathogen only in late-stage disease when the CD4 cell count is usually less than 50/mm³.

The differential diagnosis based on chest radiographic changes is summarized in Table 1.27. It is emphasized that

Table 1.26.
Pulmonary Infection

Agent	Course[a]	Frequency/Setting	Typical Findings	Diagnosis[b]	Treatment
PARASITE					
Pneumocystis[c]	Subacute or chronic	Very common in late stages of HIV infection (CD4 <200; median CD4-100 without prophylaxis, 30 with prophylaxis)	Interstitial infiltrates; negative radiograph in 10%–30%; atypical lobe findings: upper lobe infiltrates especially in patients receiving aerosolized pentamidine; also has ↑ lactate dehydrogenase (90%), ↓ pO₂ (95%), ↓ pulse oximetry, ↓ diffusing capacity	Cytopath of induced sputum or FOB; yield with induced sputum 40%–80% (average 60%) and depends on quality assurance; yield with FOB BAL: >95%	TMP-SMX Alternatives: dapsone-trimethoprim; clindamycin-primaquin; atovaquone
BACTERIA					
Streptococcus pneumoniae	Acute	Common, all stages HIV infection	Lobar or broncho-pneumonia ± pleural effusion	Sputum GS, Quellung, culture, blood culture	Penicillin Cefotaxime or ceftriaxone
Hemophilus influenzae	Acute	Moderately common; all stages HIV infection	Bronchopneumonia	Sputum GS and culture	Cefuroxime TMP-SMX

[a]Course: Acute—symptoms evolve over days; subacute—symptoms evolve over 2–6 weeks; chronic—symptoms evolve over >4 weeks.
[b]Diagnosis: Expectorated sputum for bacterial culture should have cytological screening to show predominance of PMN; Gram stain (GS) and Quellung (if GS suggest *S. pneumoniae*). Induced sputum is usually reserved for patients with nonproductive cough and suspected *P. carnii* pneumonia (PCP) or *M. tuberculosis*. Fiberoptic bronchoscoKpy (FOB) assumes bronchoalveolar lavage specimen (BAL) ± touch preparations, bronchial washings, bronchial brush, or transbronchial biopsy; the usual specimen for PCP is BAL. Detection of fungi includes stains (KOH and/or Gomori methenamine silver stain) and culture (Sabouraud's media); *Candida* sp. grow on conventional bacteria media. Detection of viruses includes cytopathology for inclusions (herpes viruses—CMV, HSV, VZV); FA for HSV and influenza; cultures are for herpes viruses and, with special request, influenza virus.

(continued)

Table 1.26. (continued)

Agent	Course[a]	Frequency/Setting	Typical Findings	Diagnosis[b]	Treatment
Gram-negative bacilli	Acute	Uncommon, except with nosocomial infection, neutropenia, cavity, chronic antibiotic exposure, or late stage disease (esp. *Pseudomonas aeruginosa*)	Lobar or bronchopneumonia, cavity	Sputum GS and culture	Aminoglycoside plus ciprofloxacin, cephalosporin or imipenem
Legionella[c]	Acute	Unusual except in epidemic areas	Bronchopneumonia multiple noncontiguous segments	Sputum DFA stain and/or culture; urinary antigen (*Legionella pneumophila*, type 1)	Erythromycin; clarithromycin; azithromycin or fluoroquinolones
VIRUS CMV	Subacute or chronic	Common isolate, rare cause of pulmonary disease; advanced HIV infection with median CD4 <20	Interstitial infiltrates	Yield of CMV by cytopathology or culture with FOB is 20%–50%; diagnosis of CMV pneumonitis requires CMV by biopsy, or CMV plus progressive disease and no alternative pathogen	Ganciclovir

(continued)

Table 1.26. (continued)

Agent	Course[a]	Frequency/Setting	Typical Findings	Diagnosis[b]	Treatment
Influenza[c]	Acute	Influenza is common; influenza pneumonia is rare; any stage of HIV infection; frequency and course similar to patients without HIV infection	Upper respiratory infection, pharyngitis, bronchitis—most common	Culture of throat washing FA stain of sputum serology, epidemiology in community and typical symptoms	Amantidine (influenza type A)
HSV, VZV, RSV, paraflu	Acute	Rare causes of pneumonia	Bronchopneumonia, interstitial infiltrates are rare except with bacterial super-infection Diffuse or nodular pneumonia, bronchopneumonia	Culture of sputum or FOB commonly yields HSV as a contaminant from upper airways	HSV—acyclovir
Mycobacterium tuberculosis (MTB)[c]	Chronic, subacute, or asymptomatic	Moderate ↑ IVDA, urban areas; all stages—mean CD4 is 200–300/mm³, extrapulmonary TB common	Variable; focal infiltrates, reticular, cavity disease, hilar adenopathy, lower and middle lobe involvement common, pleural effusion	Sputum AFB stain and culture; induced sputum or bronchoscopy	INH, rifampin, PZA plus ethambutol or streptomycin

Detection of these organisms in respiratory secretions is essentially diagnostic of disease; other organisms may be contaminants, colonizing mucosal surfaces, or commensals.

CMV, cytomegalovirus; FA, fluorescent antibody; HSV, herpes simplex virus; INH, isoniazide; IVDA, injection drug user; LP, lumbar puncture; PZA, purazinamide; RSV, respiratory syncytial virus; VZV, varicella zoster.

(continued)

81

Table 1.26. *(continued)*

Agent	Course[a]	Frequency/Setting	Typical Findings	Diagnosis[b]	Treatment
M. avium	Chronic	Moderate (see diagnosis); CD4 <50	Variable	Recovery in sputum or FOB: must distinguish from MTB (DNA or radiometric culture)	Clarithromycin plus ethambutol ± rifabutin or ciprofloxacin
Fungi Cryptococcus	Chronic, subacute, or asymptomatic	Moderately common: advanced HIV infection; with median CD4 of 50; 80% have cryptococcal meningitis	Nodule, cavity, diffuse, or nodular infiltrates	Sputum or FOB stain and culture; serum cryptococcal antigen; LP indicated analysis	Fluconazole or amphotericin B
Histoplasma capsulatum[c]	Chronic or subacute	Uncommon outside endemic area; usually advanced HIV infection with disseminated histoplasmosis—median CD4 is 50	Diffuse or nodular infiltrates, nodule, focal infiltrate, cavity, hilar adenopathy	Sputum or FOB stain and culture; serum and urine antigen assay; serology; highest yield with culture: marrow	Amphotericin B, then itraconazole

(continued)

Table 1.26. (continued)

Agent	Course[a]	Frequency Setting	Typical Findings	Diagnosis[b]	Treatment
Aspergillus	Acute or subacute	Up to 4% of patients with advanced HIV infection; corticosteroids and neutropenia (ANC <500/mm³) predispose	Focal infiltrate, cavity often pleural-based	Sputum stain and culture: false-positive and false-negative cultures common; most reliable are positive stain in typical setting or biopsy evidence of tissue invasion	Amphotericin B or itraconazole
Miscellaneous Kaposi's sarcoma	Chronic or asymptomatic	Moderately common in patients with cutaneous Kaposi's sarcoma	Interstitial, alveolar, or nodular infiltrates; hilar adenopathy pleural effusions; gallium scan usually negative	FOB: endobronchial lesion often seen; yield with FOB biopsy of parenchymal lesion is only 10%–30%	Chemotherapy
Lymphoma	Chronic or asymptomatic	Uncommon, but may be presenting site	Interstitial, alveolar, or nodular infiltrates; cavity, hilar adenopathy, pleural effusions	FOB: yield very poor; open lung biopsy usually required	Chemotherapy

83

Table 1.27
Differential Diagnosis of Pulmonary Complications Based on Radiographic Findings

DIFFUSE RETICULONODULAR

INFILTRATES

Pneumocystis carinii
P. carinii + cytomegalovirus
Miliary tuberculosis
Histoplasmosis
Coccidioidomycosis
Kaposi's sarcoma
Lymphocytic interstitial pneumonia
Leishmania donovani
Toxoplasma gondii

NODULES

Mycobacterium tuberculosis
Cryptococcosis
Kaposi's sarcoma

CONSOLIDATION

Common
Pyogenic bacteria
Cryptococcosis
Kaposi's sarcoma

Rare
Nocardia
M. tuberculosis
M. kansasii
Bordatella bronchiseptica

PLEURAL EFFUSION

Common
Pyogenic bacteria
Kaposi's sarcoma
M. tuberculosis
Cryptococcosis
P. carinii
Hypoalbuminemia
Septic emboli (IDU)
Heart failure
Aspergillosis

Rare
Rhodococcus equi
Histoplasmosis
Coccidioidomycosis
Leishmania donovani
Lymphoma
M. avium
Nocardia
P. carinii

(continued)

Table 1.27 (continued)

HILAR ADENOPATHY

M. tuberculosis
Cryptococcosis
M. avium
Histoplasmosis
Coccidioidomycosis
Kaposi's sarcoma
Lymphoma

NORMAL

P. carinii
M. tuberculosis
Cryptococcus
M. avium

CAVITARY DISEASE

Common	Rare
Gram-negative bacilli	Legionella
M. tuberculosis	P. carinii
M. kansasii	Aspergillus
Cryptococcosis	P. aeruginosa
Histoplasmosis	Lymphoma
Coccidioidomycosis	M. avium
Rhodococcus equi	
Anaerobic bacteria	
S. aureus (IDU)	

IDU, injection drug user.

PCP is one of the few forms of pneumonitis in which a chest radiograph is reportedly normal in 10%–20% of cases, and, in some series, up to 40% of cases (5). Tuberculosis may also be found in expectorated sputum samples in patients who have completely normal chest radiographs as well.

Diagnostic evaluation. Diagnostic testing depends to some extent on the resources available and on the diagnostic probabilities. Production of expectorated sputum as a prominent feature of the infection is evidence against PCP, and these specimens should be processed with conventional laboratory methods with stain and culture for bacteria, fungi, and *Mycobacteria*. Patients who do not have a productive cough, but complain of progressive fever and dyspnea, need to be evaluated for PCP if the CD4 cell count is less than 300/mm^3. The usual tests are blood gases to detect hypoxemia; some authorities advocate gallium scans or pulmonary function tests to measure CO diffusing capacity. The serum lactate dehydrogenase (LDH) is elevated in over 90% of patients, but is considered a nonspecific finding. Patients with diffuse interstitial infiltrates or a negative chest radiograph with hypoxemia and typical symptoms need to be evaluated and/or treated for PCP.

The preferred diagnostic test for PCP is fiberoptic bronchoscopy, which has a sensitivity of 95% and specificity of 100%. Many clinics and hospitals offer induced sputum as an alternative screening test; the yield with this specimen source is highly variable but averages about 60% when there is careful quality control (173). An argument may be made for empiric treatment of patients with atypical presentation to avoid the cost and discomfort of induced sputum or bronchoscopy. This is actually considered cost-effective when there is typical presentation. However, a confirmed diagnosis is clearly preferred in patients who are seriously ill, for patients given corticosteroid therapy for a

pO_2 less than 70 mm Hg, and for patients with atypical presentations.

Acid-fast stains should be done in all patients with suspected pulmonary tuberculosis. The suspected diagnosis of pulmonary TB should be substantially higher in patients with HIV infection owing to the high prevalence of TB and also to the fact that many have an atypical presentation, including lower lobe infiltrates, the lack of cavity formation, and false-negative purified protein derivative (PPD) skin tests. The sensitivity of expectorated sputum AFB among patients with positive cultures is about 60%. Some who have positive AFB stains have MOTT, primarily *M. avium* or *M. kansasii,* but *M. tuberculosis* accounts for the great majority of positive AFB smears in HIV-infected patients, even in low prevalence areas for TB.

THERAPY

As with all pneumonias, therapeutic decisions are remarkably simplified if an etiologic diagnosis is established. Guidelines are summarized in Table 1.26.

For patients with no established diagnosis, therapeutic decisions are based on probabilities according to clinical presentation, CD4 cell count as an indicator of stage of disease, changes on radiograph, and severity of illness. General principles are as follows.

1. Patients with diffuse, bilateral interstitial infiltrates and a low CD4 cell count must be treated for PCP. The preferred drug is trimethoprim-sulfamethoxazole owing to established merit and activity against many bacterial pathogens as well. Alternative regimens (pentamidine, dapsone-trimethoprim, clindamycin-primaquine, atovaquone, and trimetrexate) have established merit for PCP, but lack activity against any other pathogens; if bacterial infection is considered possible or probable it is common practice to add an antibacterial agent such as a cephalosporin.

2. Patients with focal pneumonia and an acute presentation regardless of stage of disease need to be treated for pneumococcal pneumonia and many should be treated for other bacterial agents as well. The selection of agents is often facilitated by Gram stain and culture of expectorated sputum. Guidelines are summarized in Tables 1.9 and 1.11.

3. Patients with cavitary disease need to be assessed for TB and other *Mycobacteria,* anaerobic bacteria, nocardia, PCP, pathogenic fungi, cryptococcus, and *R. equi;* the usual empiric selection often includes four agents for TB pending cultures while the diagnostic evaluation is being done. This diagnosis is far more plausible with a history of a cough 1 month or more and less than 1 year. When hospitalized, such patients should be managed with appropriate precautions for TB. The major cause of lung abscess in AIDS patients is aerobic GNB, and these are easily detected in respiratory secretions of most patients (174).

Aspiration Pneumonia

DEFINITION

Aspiration pneumonia refers to the pulmonary sequelae resulting from abnormal entry of endogenous secretions or exogenous substances into the lower airways. There are two requirements: First, a breakdown of the usual defenses that protect the tracheobronchial tree such as glottic closure, cough reflex, and other clearing mechanisms of the lower respiratory tract; second, pulmonary complications.

INCIDENCE

Most studies of community-acquired pneumonia indicate that aspiration pneumonia accounts for 5%–10% of cases (9,75–86). The appellation CAP is generally applied to patients who have a predisposing condition to aspiration, a chest radiograph showing involvement of a dependent pulmonary segment, and the lack of a likely pulmonary pathogen with aerobic cultures of expectorated sputum. Many of these patients have infections involving anaerobic bacteria, which are not detected with the usual diagnostic methods in current use. Studies using transtracheal aspiration to define the infecting flora suggest that anaerobes are involved in 20%–30% of cases of CAP, suggesting that aspiration pneumonia involving these organisms may be more frequent than generally suspected (95,96). Patients with nosocomial pneumonia are frequently prone to aspiration, which is a frequent pathophysiologic mechanism for bacteria to reach the lower airways, and anaerobes are found in up to 30% of nosocomial pneumonias (139). Nevertheless, most of these cases involving anaerobes also involve GNB or *S. aureus* as well, and these latter organisms are probably far more important in terms of therapeutic decisions.

PREDISPOSING CONDITIONS

Numerous studies indicate that even healthy persons periodically aspirate, but the aspiratory event usually passes without recognition and without detectable sequelae. The decisive factor in the development of pulmonary complications relates to the frequency, volume, and character of the material aspirated. Conditions associated with an increased incidence of aspiration are summarized in Table 1.28 and include *a)* reduced levels of consciousness; *b)* dysphagia from neurologic deficits or diseases of the esophagus; *c)* mechanical disruption of the glottic closure or cardiac sphincter due to tracheostomy, endotracheal tubes, or nasogastric feeding tubes; *d)* anatomic abnormalities including tracheoesophageal fistulas, esophageal strictures, diverticuli or gastric outlet obstruction, or *e)* pharyngeal anesthesia.

Table 1.28
Conditions that Predispose to Aspiration

Altered consciousness
  Alcoholism, seizures, cerebrovascular accident, head
    trauma, general anesthesia, drug overdose
Dysphagia
  Esophageal disorder: stricture, neoplasm, diverticular, tra-
    cheoesophageal fistula, incompetent cardiac sphincter
Gastroesophageal reflux
Neurologic disorder
  Multiple sclerosis, Parkinson's disease, myasthenia gravis,
    pseudobulbar palsy
Mechanical disruption of the usual defense barriers
  Nasogastric tube, endotracheal intubation, tracheostomy,
    upper gastrointestinal endoscopy
Protracted vomiting
Pharyngeal anesthesia

CLASSIFICATION

Aspiration pneumonia refers to at least three distinctive
syndromes based on the character of the inoculum that de-
fines the pathogenesis of pulmonary complications, clinical
presentation, and treatment as summarized in Table 1.29
(175).

Chemical pneumonitis. Chemical pneumonitis refers to
fluids that are inherently toxic to the lungs and lower
airways that can initiate an inflammatory reaction inde-
pendent of bacterial infection. Examples include acid
(especially gastric acid), volatile hydrocarbons (gasoline,
kerosene), animal fats, mineral oil, and alcohol. The best
studied of these is chemical pneumonitis due to gastric acid
as classically described by Mendelson in 1946 and often
referred to as "Mendelson's syndrome" (176,177). This is
a rapidly evolving syndrome with symptoms developing

Table 1.29

Classification of Aspiration Pneumonia

Inoculum	Pulmonary Sequelae	Clinical Features	Therapy
Acid	Chemical pneumonitis	Acute dyspnea, tachypnea tachycardia; ± cyanosis, bronchospasm, fever Sputum: pink, frothy Radiograph: infiltrates in one or both lower lobes Hypoxemia	Positive pressure breathing Intravenous fluids Tracheal suction
Oropharyngeal bacteria	Bacterial infection	Usually insidious onset Cough, fever, purulent sputum Radiograph: infiltrate involving dependent pulmonary segment or lobe ± cavitation	Antibiotics
Inert fluids	Mechanical obstruction Reflex airway closure	Acute dyspnea, cyanosis ± apnea Pulmonary edema	Tracheal suction Intermittent positive pressure breathing with oxygen and isoproterenol
Particulate matter	Mechanical obstruction	Dependent on level of obstruction, ranging from acute apnea and rapid death to irritating chronic cough ± recurrent infections	Extraction of particulate matter Antibiotics for superimposed infection

within 2 hours of the aspiration event. The cardinal features of the disease include acute illness with precipitous onset of respiratory distress following aspiration. Within minutes of aspiration, chest radiographs invariably show an infiltrate located in one or both lower lobes with mottled densities.

Clinical features include fever; many patients have bronchospasm and arterial hypoxemia is nearly always present; most patients have an abrupt onset and nearly all are aspiration-prone with compromised consciousness or dysphagia. The subsequent course follows one of three patterns: some patients have a fulminant course that progresses rapidly to the acute respiratory distress syndrome (ARDS). A second pattern is rapid improvement with radiograph clearing in a mean time of 4.5 days. Third is a group of patients who have initial improvement, but then deteriorate owing to a pulmonary superinfection (178).

Studies of gastric acid pneumonitis in animals indicates two requirements: First, a pH of 2.5 or less and, second, a relatively large inoculum (179). The diagnosis is usually made presumptively based on clinical observations, chest radiograph, and blood gas studies. A highly characteristic feature is the rapid evolution, which is sometimes compared to a flash burn of the lung. Bronchoscopy is often done in these patients to remove particulate matter, which often demonstrates erythema of the bronchi, indicating acute injury.

Treatment includes intravenous fluid support using colloids to restore circulating volume and osmotic pressure, and positive-pressure ventilation. It was once common practice to use corticosteroids, but clinical studies as well as animal experiments show that this tactic is unsuccessful and not indicated. In fact, one study showed that these agents predispose to superinfection with GNB (180). Antimicrobial agent use is controversial. No evidence exists that bacteria play any role in the initial events, although it is often difficult to exclude bacterial infection and the acid-injured lung is prone to infection so that some would use this for prophylaxis. Nevertheless, there is no evidence that these drugs alter clinical outcome and there is the inherent danger of promoting infection by relatively resistant bacteria (181).

Mechanical obstruction. The second category of aspiration pneumonia is the sequelae of aspirating fluids or particulate matter resulting in mechanical obstruction. The fluids are those that are not inherently toxic to the lung, but the failure to clear them may cause interference with air exchange. Examples are saline, barium, water, and gastric contents with a pH exceeding 2.5. One example of this type of aspiration pneumonia is the drown victim. Another is the patient who aspirates relatively large volumes, but lacks the cough reflex necessary for clearance owing to coma or severe neurologic impairment. The obvious critical therapeutic modality is tracheal suction. If a subsequent radiograph shows no pulmonary infiltrate, no therapy is required except for efforts to prevent similar episodes in the future.

The most frequent solid particles aspirated are peanuts, other vegetable particles, inorganic materials, and teeth. Some are radiopaque and, therefore, can be demonstrated on chest radiograph. The severity of the immediate consequences depends on the level of obstruction. Large objects that lodge in the larynx or trachea may cause sudden respiratory distress, aphonia, cyanosis, and death. Aspiration of smaller particles causes a more indolent process owing to partial or complete obstruction of smaller airways. Many patients present with cough due to bronchial irritation; dyspnea, cyanosis, unilateral wheezing, chest pain, and vomiting may be present. Chest radiographs show atelectasis or obstructive emphysema depending on the presence of complete or partial obstruction. Bacterial infection is a frequent complication so that these patients may initially present with the clinical features of a bacterial infection, usually more than 1 week after the aspiratory event, which may have passed unnoticed. Experimental studies in dogs show that bronchial occlusion is followed by infection usually involving oral anaerobic bacteria distal to the site of occlusion. Patients with this complication respond well to antibiotics, but the infection is apt to recur and recurrent pneumonia at the same anatomic site of involvement is a clue to the presence of a local lesion. The treatment of this type of mechanical obstruction includes bronchoscopy to remove the foreign particle.

Bacterial infection. The most common form of aspiration pneumonia is bacterial infection due to aspiration of bacteria that normally reside in the upper airways (38). It should be noted that many bacteria, including *S. pneumoniae, H. influenzae,* GNB, and *S. aureus,* reach the lower airways by virtue of aspiration. In these cases, the organisms are relatively virulent so that the inoculum size is small and the actual event is probably aspiration as found in relatively health hosts who are not predisposed to aspiration of large volumes.

In most cases of aspiration pneumonia, there is the predisposing condition to aspiration as summarized above; a relatively large inoculum and anaerobic bacteria are the usual pathogens. Aspiration pneumonia tends to be a more insidious process compared with acid aspiration or pneumococcal pneumonia. Radiographs generally show a pulmonary infiltrate in a dependent pulmonary segment: favored segments are the superior segment of a lower lobe or posterior segment of an upper lobe, which are dependent in the recumbent position, or in the lower lobes, which are dependent with aspiration in the upright position.

Nearly all patients will have the typical radiograph localization; many will have a relatively insidious course with fever, cough, and sputum production; about 90% will have a predisposing condition for aspiration. With anaerobic bacteria, the initial stage is pneumonitis with an infiltrate in a dependent pulmonary segment and a course that may resemble pneumococcal pneumonia or may be more indolent (182). With persistent infection exceeding 1 week, there is often progression to the late suppurative complications that include lung abscess or empyema. Characteristic features of late presentation include tissue necrosis with cavity formation and/or empyema, putrid discharge, and evidence of chronic disease with prolonged symptoms, weight loss, and anemia.

THERAPY

Preferred treatment for aspiration pneumonia involving anaerobic bacteria is clindamycin; alternative agents that are often effective include a betalactam-betalactamase inhibitor, penicillin, or amoxicillin or a combination of metronidazole plus penicillin (183–185).

PREVENTION

Recommendations to reduce or prevent aspiration are aimed at the pathophysiologic mechanisms in the predisposed host. Patients with reduced consciousness should be placed in a semi-recumbent position with the head of the bed at 45 degrees or more to reduce gastroesophageal reflux (158). Patients requiring feeding tubes should have small-bore tubes, tubes placed in the duodenum, and withholding of feedings if residual volumes exceed 30 mL. H2 blockers and antacids may be used to decrease gastric acidity to reduce chemical pneumonitis, but this invites the potential problem of bacterial overgrowth with GNB and the risk of Gram-negative bacillary pneumonia (159). Patients with endotracheal tubes should have the cuff pressure at 25 mm H_2O. Patients with gastroesophageal reflux should have the head of the bed elevated before sleep, food avoidance for several hours before sleep, weight reduction if appropriate, and antacids or H2 blockers. Metoclopramide (10 mg IV) is often used for patients undergoing emergency surgery to promote gastric emptying and improve lower esophageal sphincter tone.

Empyema

Empyema was once a relatively common complication of bacterial pneumonia, but the frequency is now reduced to less than 2% of cases (71), suggesting that antimicrobial agents have had a pronounced effect in preventing this complication.

DEFINITION

"Empyema" literally refers to pus in a body cavity, but the term is usually used synonymously with a pleural empyema. The classic definition is purulent fluid meaning "pleural pus." More recent definitions have included a pleural effusion with a leukocyte count exceeding 25,000/mL and a predominance of polymorphonuclear leukocytes, microorganisms demonstrated by stain or culture, or, most recently, a pleural fluid pH <7.1 (11).

PATHOPHYSIOLOGY

Most empyemas occur as complications of bacterial infections of the lung. The most common mechanism is direct spread from the lung infection to a parapneumonic effusion; about 20%–40% represent a complication of a bronchial-pleural fistula. The second most common mechanism of empyema is a complication of surgery, usually thoracic surgery with introduction of bacteria to the pleural space at the time of surgery or via a thoracotomy drain. Miscellaneous pathways for bacteria to reach the pleural space include bacteremic seeding, esophageal perforation, transdiaphragmatic spread from intra-abdominal infection, or chest trauma, especially when there is a hemothorax.

INCIDENCE

Empyema currently accounts for 0.5–0.8 cases per 1000 admissions (186,187). In the prepenicillin era this was noted in 10%–20% of cases of pneumococcal pneumonia (90). The frequency now is 1%–2% of community-acquired pneumonia sufficiently severe to require hospitalization (71).

BACTERIOLOGY

Studies of empyema in the pre-chemotherapeutic era show that *S. pneumoniae* consistently accounted for two thirds of cases, group A beta-hemolytic streptococci accounted for 10%–15%, and *S. aureus* accounted for 5%–8% (188). Anaerobic cultures were usually not done, but investigators reporting at that time claimed 5%–7% were noted to be "putrid." The more recent reports of empyema indicate that the microbial cause depends largely on the pathophysiology (Table 1.30) (189). The predominant pathogens in cases associated with pneumonitis with or without a lung abscess are anaerobic bacteria; *S. pneumoniae* is a relatively unusual organism accounting for only 5%–15% according to 15 reports published from 1960–1995 (186–189). Other common pathogens include *S. aureus* usually reported in 10%–40%, and Gram-negative bacteria in 25%–50%. The yield of anaerobes is dependent to a large extent on the rigor of laboratory studies and ranges from 20%–75%. Most studies indicate that 5%–20% are sterile, implying either inadequate culture techniques, erroneous diagnosis, or culture failure due to prior antibiotic usage. The frequency of polymicrobial infections is reported in 20%–70% of cases and this is the expected finding in patients with anaerobic infections. The

Table 1.30
Bacteriology of Empyema

Cases[a]	1934–1939 3000	1950–1970 1017	1970–1995 1289
Streptococcus pneumoniae	64%	5%	7%
Group A streptococci	9%	2%	1%
Staphylococcus aureus	7%	41%	15%
Gram-negative bacillus	NS	32%	15%
Anaerobes	5%	11%	19%
Mixed infection	NS	20%	25%
Sterile	NS	10%	28%

[a]Total reported cases reviewed; % is the cumulative total for designated organism expressed as a percent of the total cases.
Adapted from: Bartlett JG. Empyema. In Gorbach SL, Bartlett JG, Blacklow NR, eds. Infectious diseases. Philadelphia: WB Saunders, 1997.
NS, not significant.

bacteriology of empyema following thoracic surgery is usually GNB or *S. aureus* (189,190). Rare cases of empyema have been described with *Legionella, Salmonella, Listeria monocytogenes,* some alpha-hemolytic streptococci including *S. mitis* and *S. milleri, Eikenella, Pasteurella multicidia, Neisseria meningitidis, Actinomyces,* and *Moraxella catarrhalis.*

PRESENTATION
The usual symptoms are those of pulmonary infection including fever, cough, and sputum production. Most patients also have pleurisy, and this may be the observation that prompts medical attention. Chest radiographs show a pleural effusion; this may be found in up to 30%–40% of patients with pneumonia, but only about 3% will satisfy the definition for an empyema.

DIAGNOSIS

The diagnosis of empyema is established with appropriate studies of pleural fluid obtained by thoracentesis. It may be difficult to drain fluid if it is thick and purulent and requires a large needle; if there is a relatively small or a loculated effusion, the thoracentesis should be done with ultrasound guidance. Standard tests on pleural fluid include pH, lactic dehydrogenase, white blood cell count and differential, and appropriate stains and culture. Microbiologic studies include Gram stain and AFB stain, and culture to detect bacteria (aerobic and anaerobic cultures) and *Mycobacteria*. The diagnosis is established if there is purulent fluid, a positive culture for a likely pathogen, or a pH <7.1 (12). It should be noted that the pleural fluid pH does not establish the diagnosis of empyema by classic criteria, but it has important implications regarding management. Findings that support the diagnosis of empyema are a pleural fluid pH below 7.1, lactic dehydrogenase over 1000 IU/L, leukocyte count over 30,000/mL with a predominance of neutrophils, glucose concentration less than 60 mg/mL (or a pleural fluid: serum glucose ratio below 0.5), or a pleural fluid lactate exceeding 5 mmol/L (11,12). In most instances these tests will be mutually supporting. A meta-analysis shows that the most useful of the chemistry tests (nonbacteriologic studies) is the pleural fluid pH (12).

MICROBIOLOGY

The following observations apply to specific microbes that are noted in empyema.

Anaerobic bacteria. Anaerobic bacteria are reported in 10%–15% of empyema cases, but the frequency is probably much higher when anaerobic culture techniques are adequate. In our experience, these organisms were found in 63 of 83 patients with empyema (76%) (191). Clinical features include the presence of a pulmonary infiltrate that is often accompanied by abscess formation. Many result from a bronchopleural fistula as indicated by bubbling of drainage tubes under suction. The fluid is often extremely thick, loculated, and difficult to remove so that most patients require open surgical drainage or decortication. Many patients have putrid pleural fluid, which is considered diagnostic of infection involving anaerobes. Although most result from aspiration pneumonia, some represent extension from a subphrenic abscess.

Streptococcus pneumoniae. Parapneumonic effusions are found in 20%–50% of patients with pneumococcal pneumonia, but most are sterile effusions that resolve with standard antibiotic treatment. This organism accounted for about two thirds of all empyemas in the prepenicillin era, but now is found in only about 3%–7%. The assumption is that successful treatment of pneumococcal pneumonia prevented this late complication and this presumably accounts for the sharp drop in the frequency of empyemas and the even larger decrease in the frequency of pneumococcal empyema. In patients who have this complication, larger doses of antibiotics (such as 10–20 million units of penicillin per day for penicillin-sensitive strains) are used and treatment is continued for prolonged periods.

Streptococcal empyema. Group A beta-hemolytic streptococci is a relatively unusual cause of pneumonia. However, a prominent feature of pneumonia caused by group a beta-hemolytic streptococci is rapid accumulation of a pleural effusion with fibropurulent or hemorrhagic fluid. This is noted in up to 80% of acute pneumonias involving group A streptococci and presumably reflects a rapid migration of organisms to the pleura via lymphatic channels. Streptococci accounted for 10%–15% of all empyemas in the prepenicillin era, but are now relatively rare. It should be emphasized that there are multiple species of streptococci that may be involved in empyema; the unusual features of the clinical course summarized above apply only to those caused by group A beta-hemolytic streptococci.

Staphylococcus aureus. *Staphylococcus aureus* is a relatively common cause of empyema that most often represents a complication of thoracic surgery or empyema in infants. In adults with primary staphylococcal pneumonia, pleural fluid collections are common, but most are sterile.

TREATMENT

The usual treatment of empyema consists of antibiotics directed against the pathogen combined with drainage, which is considered critical.

Antibiotic selection is obviously simplified if there is a bacteriologic diagnosis using Gram stain and/or cultures. The presence of putrid empyema fluid is diagnostic of anaerobic infection and a Gram stain showing a polymicrobial flora is strongly suggestive. Virtually all antibiotics diffuse well into pleural fluid so that local instillation is usually not advocated.

The most difficult component of treatment is often the drainage procedure, which is dictated by the size of the effusion, loculations, stage of disease, and trial and error. Guidelines are provided in Table 1.31. With regard to stages, there are three sequential categories that merge indistinguishably, but adequate drainage becomes progressively difficult. The initial stage is the "exudative stage," which is characterized by a collection of thin, free-flowing fluid that usually contains a relatively small number of leukocytes and microorganisms. The lung at this time is readily reexpanded. The second stage is the "fibropurulent stage" with large numbers of leukocytes and a fibrin accumulation. The fibrin is deposited in both the parietal and visceral pleura at the site of involvement causing loculation and fixation of the lung. The final stage is the "organizing

Table 1.31
Classification and Therapy of Parapneumonic Effusions and Empyema[a]

Class	Diagnostic criteria	Treatment
1. Insignificant effusion	Small (<10 mm fluid on lateral decubitus film—see text)	Antibiotics Thoracentesis usually unnecessary
2. Parapneumonic effusion	>10 mm thick on lateral decubitus film	Antibiotics Thoracentesis indicated
3. Borderline complicated effusion	pH 7–7.2 and/or lactate dehydrogenase >1,000 IU/L; glucose >40 mg/dL; negative Gram stain and culture	Antibiotics and serial thoracentesis; tube thoracostomy sometimes necessary
4. Simple, complicated effusion	pH <7 and/or glucose <40 mg/dL and/or Gram stain or culture positive	Antibiotics plus tube thoracostomy
5. Complex complicated effusion	Above plus multiloculated	Antibiotics Tube thoracostomy and thrombolytics
6. Simple empyema	Pus Single loculus or free-flowing	Antibiotics Tube thoracostomy ± decortication
7. Complex empyema	Pus Multiloculated	Antibiotics Tube thoracostomy plus thrombolytics Thoracoscopy or decortication

[a]Adapted from: Sahn SA. Management of complicated parapneumonic effusions. Am Rev Respir Dis 1993;148:813.

stage" with fibroblasts that produce a pleural peel of thick, fibrous tissue. At this last stage, the empyema is regarded as chronic and the exudate consists of thick pus.

During the initial exudative phase, the empyema may resolve with antibiotic therapy for the associated pneumonia, although repeated thoracentesis or tube thoracostomy drainage may be required. The necessity for thoracostomy drainage increases with a lower pH, lower glucose level, and a higher LDH. Some authorities base the decision to perform thoracostomy in patients with nonpurulent effusions on the pleural fluid pH (see Table 1.31 (11). Thus, a pH below 7.0 will require tube drainage and those with a pH exceeding 7.3 will resolve with antibiotics alone. In the pH range of 7.0 to 7.3, some authorities use repeated thoracentesis and resort to thoracostomy only with persistent signs of sepsis after 3–4 days or rapid accumulation of fluid. A thoracostomy is required during the fibropurulent phase. In some cases, large-bore needles are required to obtain adequate drainage and there are often loculations that may require insertion of multiple tubes, sometimes facilitated by fluoroscopic, computed tomographic, or ultrasonic guidance. This type of closed drainage with suction is recommended as the initial drainage procedure when the fluid is thick, when there is evidence of a bronchopleural fistula, or when the pleural fluid is putrid. Tubes are left in place until the empyema cavity is obliterated by expansion of the lung, pleural drainage is less than 25 mL/day, the patient is afebrile, and any prior bronchopleural fistula is sealed. Failure to respond with clinical improvement in 48–72 hours usually indicates inadequate drainage, occlusion of the tube, improperly placed tube, a debilitated host, severe pneumonia, or inappropriate antibiotic selection. The adequacy of tube placement may be evaluated by a radiograph or, preferably, computed tomography.

During the organizing stage, most patients require open drainage with rib resection or decortication. Indications for these procedures are persistent signs of sepsis, failure to demonstrate adequate reduction in cavity size, or inadequate drainage despite reinsertion of tubes.

References

1. American Thoracic Society. Guidelines for the initial management of adults with community-acquired pneumonia: diagnosis, assessment of severity, and initial antimicrobial therapy. Am Rev Resp Dis 1993;148:1418.

2. The British Thoracic Society. Guidelines for the management of community-acquired pneumonia in adults admitted to hospital. Br J Hosp Med 1993;49:346.

3. Garibaldi RA. Epidemiology of community-acquired respiratory tract infections in adults: incidence, etiology, and impact. Am J Med 1985;78:32S.

4. Caldwell A, Glauser FL, Smith WR, et al. The effects of dehydration on the radiographic and pathologic appearance of experimental canine segmental pneumonia. Am Rev Respir Dis 1975;112:651.

5. Opravil M, Marincek B, Fuchs WA, et al. Shortcomings of chest radiography in detecting *Pneumocystis carinii* pneumonia. J Acquir Immune Defic Syndr Hum Retrovirol 1994;7:39.

6. Gonzales R, Sande M. What will it take to stop physicians from prescribing antibiotics in acute bronchitis? Lancet 1995; 345:665.

7. Halsey PB, Albaum MN, Li YH, et al. Do pulmonary radiographic findings at presentation predict mortality in patients with community-acquired pneumonia? Arch Intern Med 1996;156:2206.

8. Janssen RS, St. Louis ME, Statten GA, et al. HIV infection among patients in U.S. acute care hospitals: strategies for the counseling and testing of hospital patients. N Engl J Med 1992;327:445.

9. Mundy LM, Auwaerter PG, Oldach D, et al. Community-acquired pneumonia: impact of immune status. Am J Respir Crit Care Med 1995;152:1309.

10. Fine MJ, Singer DE, Hanusa BH, et al. Validation of a pneumonia prognostic index using the medisgroups comparative hospital database. Am J Med 1993;94:153.

11. Sahn SA. Management of complicated parapneumonic effusions. Am Rev Respir Dis 1993;148:813.
12. Heffner JE, Brown LK, Barbieri C, DeLeo JM. Pleural fluid chemical analysis in parapneumonic effusions. Am J Respir Crit Care Med 1995;151:1700.
13. Barrett-Conner E. The nonvalue of sputum culture in the diagnosis of pneumococcal pneumonia. Amer Rev Resp Dis 1970;103:845.
14. Fiala M. A study of the combined role of viruses, mycoplasmas and bacteria in adult pneumonias. Am J Med Sci 1969;257:44.
15. Rathbun HK, Govani I. Mouse inoculation as a means of identifying pneumococci in sputum. Johns Hopkins Med J 1967;120:46.
16. Mufson MA, Chang V, Gill V, et al. The role of viruses, mycoplasmas and bacteria in acute pneumonia in civilian adults. Am J Epidemiol 1967;86:526.
17. Murray PR, Washington JA, II. Microscopic and bacteriologic analysis of expectorated sputum. Mayo Clin Proc 1975;50:339.
18. Jefferson H, Dalton HP, Escobar MR, Allison MJ. Transportation delay and the microbiological quality of clinical specimens. Am J Clin Pathol 1975;64:689.
19. Fekety FR Jr, Caldwell J, Gump D, et al. Bacteria, viruses and mycoplasmas in acute pneumonia in adults. Am Rev Respir Dis 1971;104:499.
20. Geckler RW, Gremillion DH, McAllister CK, et al. Microscopic and bacteriological comparison of paired sputa and transtracheal aspirates. J Clin Microbiol 1977;6:396.
21. Van Scoy RE. Bacterial sputum cultures: a clinician's viewpoint. Mayo Clin Pract 1977;52:39.
22. Fine MJ, Orloff JJ, Rihs JD, et al. Evaluation of housestaff physicians' preparation and interpretation of sputum gram stains for community-acquired pneumonia. J Gen Intern Med 1991;6:189.
23. Gleckman R, DeVita J, Hibert D, et al. Sputum gram stain assessment in community-acquired bacteremic pneumonia. J Clin Microbiol 1988;26:846.
24. Boerner DF, Zwadyk P. The value of the sputum gram's stain in community-acquired pneumonia. JAMA 1982;247:642.
25. Kalin M, Lindberg AA, Tunevall G. Etiological diagnosis of bacterial pneumonia by gram stain and quantitative culture of expectorates. Scand J Infect Dis 1983;15:153.

26. Dans P, Charache PC, Fahey M, et al. Management of pneumonia in the prospective payment era. Arch Intern Med 1984;144:1392.

27. Spencer RC, Philip JR. Effect of previous antimicrobial therapy on bacteriological findings in patients with primary pneumonia. Lancet 1973;2:349.

28. Bartlett JG, Finegold SM. Bacteriology of expectorated sputum with quantitative culture and wash technique compared to transtracheal aspirates. Am Rev Respir Dis 1978;117:1019.

29. Wimberly N, Faling J, Bartlett JG. A fiberoptic bronchoscopy technique to obtain uncontaminated lower airway secretions for bacterial culture. Am Rev Respir Dis 1979;119;337.

30. Pecora DV, Yegian D. Bacteriology of lower respiratory tract in health and chronic disease. N Engl J Med 1958;258:71.

31. Bartlett JG. Diagnostic accuracy of transtracheal aspiration bacteriology. Am Rev Respir Dis 1977;115:777.

32. Bartlett JG. The technique of transtracheal aspiration. Journal of Critical Illness 1986;1(1):43.

33. Hahn HH, Beaty HN. Transtracheal aspiration in the evaluation of patients with pneumonia. Ann Intern Med 1970;72:183.

34. Pecora DV. How well does transtracheal aspiration reflect pulmonary infection? Chest 1974;66:220.

35. Hoeprich PD. Etiologic diagnosis of lower respiratory tract infections. California Medicine 1970;112:1.

36. Bartlett JG, Rosenblatt SM, Finegold SM. Percutaneous transtracheal aspiration in the diagnosis of anaerobic pulmonary infection. Ann Intern Med 1973;79:535.

37. Bartlett JG. Bacteriologic diagnosis in anaerobic pleuropulmonary infections. Clin Infect Dis 1993;16(Suppl 4):S443.

38. Bartlett JG. Anaerobic infections of the lung and pleural space. Clin Infect Dis 1993;16(Suppl 4):S248.

39. Bullowa JGM. The reliability of sputum typing and its relation to serum therapy. JAMA 1935;105:1512.

40. Brandt PO, Bank N, Castellino RA. Needle diagnosis of pneumonia: value in high risk patients. JAMA 1972;220:1578.

41. Bartlett JG. Invasive diagnostic techniques in pulmonary infections. In: Pennington JE, ed. Respiratory infections: diagnosis and management, 3rd ed. New York: Raven Press, 1994;73–99.

42. Herman PG, Hessel SJ. The diagnostic accuracy and complications of closed lung biopsies. Radiology 1977;125:11.

43. American Thoracic Society. Guidelines for percutaneous transthoracic needle aspiration. Am Rev Respir Dis

1989;140:255.

44. Bartlett JG, Alexander J, Mayhew J, et al. Should fiberoptic bronchoscopy aspirates be cultured? Am Rev Respir Dis 1976;114:73.

45. American Thoracic Society. Clinical role of bronchoalveolar lavage in adults with pulmonary disease. Am Rev Respir Dis 1990;142:481.

46. Murray JF, Felton CP, Garay SM, et al. Pulmonary complications of the acquired immunodeficiency syndrome. N Engl J Med 1984;310:1682.

47. Jett JR, Cortese DA, Dines DE. The value of bronchoscopy in the diagnosis of mycobacterial disease. Chest 1981;80:575.

48. Wimberly N, Willey S, Sullivan N, et al. Antibacterial properties of lidocaine. Chest 1979;76:37.

49. Wimberly NW, Bass JB, Boyd BW, et al. Use of a bronchoscopic protected catheter brush for the diagnosis of pulmonary infections. Chest 1982;81:556.

50. Dreyfuss D, Mier L, Bolurdelles G, et al. Clinical significance of borderline quantitative protected brush specimen culture results. Am Rev Respir Dis 1993;147:946.

51. Chastre J, Fagon JY, Lamer CH. Procedures for the diagnosis of pneumonia in ICU patients. Intensive Care Med 1992;18:S10.

52. Middleton R, Broughton WA, Kirkpatrick MB. Comparison of four methods for assessing airway bacteriology in intubated mechanically ventilated patients. Am J Med Sci 1992;304:239.

53. Kirkpatrick MB, Bass JB. Quantitative bacterial cultures of bronchoalveolar lavage fluids and protected brush catheter specimens from normal subjects. Am Rev Respir Dis 1989;139:546.

54. Torres A. Accuracy of diagnostic tools for the management of nosocomial respiratory infections in mechanically ventilated patients. Eur Respir J 1991;4:1010.

55. Pollock HM, Hawkins EL, Bonner JR, et al. Diagnosis of bacterial pulmonary infections during quantitative protected catheter cultures obtained during bronchoscopy. J. Clin Microbiol 1983;17:255.

56. Teague RB, Wallace RJ Jr, Awe RJ. The use of quantitative sterile brush culture and gram stain analysis in the diagnosis of lower respiratory tract infection. Chest 1981;79:157.

57. Meduri GU, Beals DH, Maijub AG, et al. Protected bronchoalveolar lavage. Am Rev Respir Dis 1991;143:855.

58. Chastre J, Fagon J-Y, Trouillet JL. Diagnosis and treatment of nosocomial pneumonia in patients in intensive care units. Clin Infect Dis 1995;21(Suppl 3):S226.
59. Meduri GU, Chastre J. The standardization of bronchoscopic techniques for ventilator-associated pneumonia. Chest 1992:102(Suppl 1):557S.
60. Chastre J, Fagon JY, Bornet M, et al. Evaluation of bronchoscopic techniques for the diagnosis of nosocomial pneumonia. Am Rev Respir Dis 1995;152:231.
61. Torres A, El-Ebiary M, Padro L, et al. Validation of different techniques for the diagnosis of ventilator-associated pneumonia. Am J Respir Crit Care Med 1994;149:324.
62. Suratt PM, Smiddy JF, Gruber B. Deaths and complications associated with fiberoptic bronchoscopy. Chest 1976;747.
63. Pereira W, Kovnat DM, Khan MA, et al. Fever and pneumonia after flexible bronchoscopy. Am Rev Respir Dis 1975;112:59.
64. Salzman SH, Schindel ML, Aranda CP, et al. The role of bronchoscopy in the diagnosis of pulmonary tuberculosis in patients at risk for HIV infection. Chest 1992;102:143.
65. Royat E, Garcia RL, Skolom J. Diagnosis of *Pneumocystis carinii* pneumonia by cytologic examination of bronchial washings. JAMA 1985;254:1950.
66. Shelhamer JH, Toews GB, Masur H, et al. Respiratory disease in the immunosuppressed patient. Ann Intern Med 1992;117:415.
67. Fagon JY, Chastre J, Hance AJ. Detection of nosocomial lung infection in ventilated patients. Am Rev Respir Dis 1988;138:110.
68. Niederman MS, Torres A, Summer W. Invasive diagnostic testing is not needed routinely to manage suspected ventilator-associated pneumonia. Am J Respir Crit Care Med 1994;150:565.
69. Chastre J, Fagon JY. Invasive diagnostic testing should be routinely used to manage ventilated patients with suspected pneumonia. Am J Respir Crit Care Med 1994;150:570.
70. Fine MJ, Auble TE, Yealy DM, et al. A prediction rule to identify low-risk patients with community-acquired pneumonia. N Engl J Med 1997;336:243.
71. Fine MJ, Smith MA, Carson CA, et al. Prognosis and outcomes of patients with community-acquired pneumonia. JAMA 1995;274:134.
72. Centers for Disease Control. Pneumonia and influenza death rates—United States, 1979–1994. MMWR 1995;44:535.

73. Fine MJ, Smith DN, Singer DE. Hospitalization decision in patients with community-acquired pneumonia: a prospective cohort study. Am J Med 1990;89:713.

74. Bartlett JG, Mundy L. Community-acquired pneumonia. N Engl J Med 1995;333:1618.

75. Opravil M, Marincek B, Fuchs WA, et al. Shortcomings of chest radiography in detecting *Pneumocystis carinii* pneumonia. J Acquir Immune Defic Syndr Hum Retrovirol 1994;7:39.

76. Mufson MA, Chang V, Gill V, et al. The role of viruses, mycoplasmas and bacteria in acute pneumonia in civilian adults. Am J Epidemiol 1967;86:526.

77. Sullivan RJ Jr, Dowdle WR, Marine WM, et al. Adult pneumonia in a general hospital: etiology and host risk factors. Arch Intern Med 1972;129:935.

78. Bisno AL, Griffin JR, Van Epps KA, et al. Pneumonia and Hong Kong influenza: a prospective study of the 1968–1969 epidemic. Am J Med Sci 1971;261:251.

79. Dorff GJ, Rytel MW, Farmer SG, et al. Etiologies and characteristic features of pneumonias in a municipal hospital. Am J Med Sci 1973;266:349.

80. Fick RB Jr, Reynolds HY. Changing spectrum of pneumonia—news media creation or clinical reality? Am J Med 1983;74:1.

81. Larsen RA, Jacobson JA. Diagnosis of community-acquired pneumonia: experience at a community hospital. Compr Ther 1984;10(43):20.

82. Marrie TJ, Durant H, Yates L. Community-acquired pneumonia requiring hospitalization: a 5 year prospective study. Rev Infect Dis 1989;11:586.

83. Farr BM, Sloman AJ, Fisch MJ. Predicting death in patients hospitalized for community-acquired pneumonia. Ann Intern Med 1991;115:428.

84. Bates JH, Campbell GD, Barron AL, et al. Microbial etiology of acute pneumonia in hospitalized patients. Chest 1992;101:1005.

85. Fang GD, Fine M, Orloff J, et al. New and emerging etiologies for community-acquired pneumonia with implication for therapy; a prospective multicenter study of 359 cases. Medicine (Baltimore) 1990;69:307.

86. Lim I, Shaw DR, Stanley DP, et al. A prospective hospital study of the aetiology of community-acquired pneumonia. Med J Aust 1989;151:87.

87. Marston BJ, Plouffe JF, Breiman RF, et al. Preliminary findings in a community-based pneumonia incidence study. In: Barbaree

JM, Breiman RF, Dufour AP, eds. Washington, DC: American Society of Microbiology, 1993;36–37.

88. Research Committee of the British Thoracic Society and the Public Health Laboratory Service. Community-acquired pneumonia in adults in British hospitals in 1982-1983: a survey of aetiology, mortality, prognostic factors and outcome. QJM 1987;239:195.

89. Fine MJ, Smith MA, Carson, et al. Prognosis and outcomes of patients with community-acquired pneumonia. JAMA 1996;275:134.

90. Heffron R. Pneumonia. Cambridge, MA: Harvard University Press, 1939.

91. Bullowa JGM. The reliability of sputum typing and its relation to serum therapy. JAMA 1935;105:1512.

92. Schreiner A, Digranes A, Myking O. Transtracheal aspiration in the diagnosis of lower respiratory tract infections. Scand J Infect Dis 1972;4:49.

93. Farr BM, Kaiser DL, Harrison BDW, et al. Prediction of microbial aetiology at admission to hospital for pneumonia from the presenting clinical features. Thorax 1989;44:1031.

94. Bartlett JG. Anaerobic bacterial pneumonitis. Am Rev Respir Dis 1979;119:19.

95. Ries K, Levison ME, Daye D. Transtracheal aspiration in pulmonary infection. Arch Intern Med 1974;133:453.

96. Pollock HM, Hawkins EL, Bonner JR, et al. Diagnosis of bacterial pulmonary infections during quantitative protected catheter cultures obtained during bronchoscopy. J. Clin Microbiol 1983;17:255.

97. Chanock RM, Mufson MA, Vloom HH, et al. Eaton agent pneumonia. JAMA 1961;175:213.

98. Finland M, Peterson OL, Allen HE, et al. Cold agglutinins. I. Occurrence of cold isohaemagglutinins in various conditions. J Clin Invest 1945;24:451.

99. Eaton MD, Meikeljohn G, van Herick W. Studies on the etiology of primary atypical pneumonia: a filterable agent transmissible to cotton rats, hamsters and chick embryos. J Exp Med 1944;79:649.

100. Foy HM. Infections caused by Mycoplasma pneumoniae and possible carrier state in a different population of patients. Clin Infect Dis 1993;17(Suppl):S37.

101. Taylor-Robinson D. Infections due to species of Mycoplasma and Ureaplasma: an update. Clin Infect Dis 1996;23:671.

102. Marston BJ, Lipman HB, Breiman RF. Surveillance for Legionnaires' disease. Arch Intern Med 1994;154:2417.
103. Edelstein PH. Legionnaires' disease. Clin Infect Dis 1993;16:741.
104. Ramirez JA, Ahkee S, Tolentino, et al. Diagnosis of *Legionella pneumophila, Mycoplasma pneumoniae,* or *Chlamydia pneumoniae* lower respiratory infection using the polymerase chain reaction on a single throat swab specimen. Diagn Microbiol Infect Dis 1996;24:7.
105. Gaydos CA, Eiden JJ, Oldach D, et al. Diagnosis of Chlamydia *pneumoniae* infection in patients with community-acquired pneumonia by polymerase chain reaction enzyme immunoassay. Clin Infect Dis 1994;19:157.
106. Grayston JT, Campbell LA, Kuo C-C, et al. A new respiratory tract pathogen: *Chlamydia* pneumoniae strain TWAR. J Infect Dis 1990;161:618.
107. Louria DB, Blumenfeld HL, Ellis JT, et al. Studies on influenza in the pandemic of 1957-1958. II. Pulmonary complications of influenza. J Clin Invest 1959;38:213.
108. Ellenbogen C, Graybill JR, Silva J, et al. Bacterial pneumonia complicating adenoviral pneumonia: a comparison of respiratory tract bacterial culture sources and effectiveness of chemoprophylaxis against bacterial pneumonia. Am J Med 1974;56:169.
109. Wenzel RP, McCormick DP, Bean WE Jr. Parainfluenza pneumonia in adults. JAMA 1972;221:294.
110. Centers for Disease Control. Parainfluenza outbreaks in extended care facilities—United States. MMWR 1978;27:475.
111. Falsey AR, Treanor JJ, Betts RF, et al. Viral respiratory infections in the institutionalized elderly: clinical and epidemiologic findings. J Am Geriatr Soc 1992;40:115.
112. Dowell SF, Anderson LJ, Gary HE Jr, et al. Respiratory syncytial virus is an important cause of community-acquired lower respiratory infection among hospitalized adults. J Infect Dis 1996;174:456.
113. Vikerfors T, Grandien M, Olcen P. Respiratory syncytial virus infections in adults. Am Rev Respir Dis 1987;136:561.
114. Doern GV, Brueggemann A, Holley HP Jr, et al. Antimicrobial resistance of *Streptococcus pneumoniae* recovered from outpatients in the United States during the winter months of 1994 to 1995: results of a 30-center national surveillance study. Antimicrob Agents Chemother 1996;40:1208.

115. Hofmann J, Cetron MS, Farley MM, et al. The prevalence of drug-resistant *Streptococcus pneumoniae* in Atlanta. N Engl J Med 1995;333:481.

116. Austrian R. Confronting drug-resistant pneumococci. Ann Intern Med 1994;121:807.

117. Gold HS, Moellering RC Jr. Antimicrobial-drug resistance. Drug Therapy 1996;335:1445.

118. Butler JC, Hofmann J, Cetron MS, et al. The continued emergence of drug-resistance *Streptococcus pneumoniae* in the United States: an update from the Centers for Disease Control and Prevention's pneumococcal sentinel surveillance system. J Infect Dis 1996;174:986.

119. Pallares R, Linares J, Vadillo M, et al. Resistance to penicillin and cephalosporin and mortality from severe pneumococcal pneumonia in Barcelona, Spain. N Engl J Med 1995;333:474.

120. Bartlett JG. IDCP Guidelines: lower respiratory tract infections. Infect Dis Clinc Pract 1996;5:147.

121. Mittl RL Jr, Schwab RJ, Duchin JS, et al. Radiographic resolution of community-acquired pneumonia. Am J Respir Crit Care Med 1994;149:630.

122. Austrian R, Winston AL. The efficacy of penicillin V in the treatment of mild or moderately severe pneumococcal pneumonia. Am J Med Sci 1956;232:624.

123. Jay SJ, Johanson WG, Pierce AK. The radiographic resolution of *Streptococcus pneumoniae* pneumonia. N Engl J Med 1975;293:798.

124. Austrian R, Gold J. Pneumococcal bacteremia with especial reference to bacteremic pneumococcal pneumonia. Ann Intern Med 1964;60:759.

125. Wheeler JH, Fishman EK. Computed tomography in the management of chest infections: current status. Clin Infect Dis 1996;23:232.

126. Craven DE, Steger KA, Barber TW. Preventing nosocomial pneumonia: state of the art and perspectives for the 1990s. Am J Med 1991;91:44S.

127. Fagon JY, Chastre J, Hance AJ, et al. Detection of nosocomial lung infection in ventilated patients: use of a protected specimen brush and quantitative culture techniques in 147 patients. Am Rev Respir Dis 1988;138:110.

128. Johanson WG, Pierce AK, Sanford JP. Changing pharyngeal

bacterial flora of hospitalized patients: emergence of gram-negative bacilli. N Engl J Med 1969;281:1137.

129. Fuxench-Lopez Z, Ramirez-Ronda CH. Pharyngeal flora in ambulatory alcoholic patients. Arch Intern Med 1978;138:1815.

130. Johanson WG Jr, Pierce AK, Sanford JP, et al. Nosocomial respiratory infections with gram-negative bacilli. The significance of colonization of the respiratory tract. Ann Intern Med 1972;77:701.

131. Mackowiak PA, Martin RM, Jones SR, et al. Pharyngeal colonization by gram-negative bacilli in aspiration-prone persons. Arch Intern Med 1978;138:1224.

132. Ramirez-Ronda CH, Fuxench-Lopez Z, Nevarez M. Increased pharyngeal bacterial colonization during viral illness. Arch Intern Med 1981;141:1599.

133. LeFrock JL, Ellis CA, Weinstein L. The relation between aerobic fecal and oropharyngeal microflora in hospitalized patients. Am J Med Sci 1979;227:275.

134. Johanson WG Jr, Woods DE, Chaudhuri T. Association of respiratory tract colonization with adherence of gram-negative bacilli to epithelial cells. J Infect Dis 1979;139:667.

135. Woods DE, Straus DC, Johanson WG Jr, et al. Role of salivary protease activity in adherence of gram-negative bacilli to mammalian buccal epithelial cells in vivo. J Clin Invest 1981;68:1435.

136. Rouby JJ, Martin de Lassale E, Poete P, et al. Nosocomial bronchopneumonia in the critically ill. Histologic and bacteriologic aspects. Am Rev Respir Dis 1992;146:1059.

137. Horan TC, White JW, Jarvis WR, et al. Nosocomial infection surveillance. MMWR 1986;35:17SS.

138. Schleupner CJ, Cobb DK. A study of the etiologies and treatment of nosocomial pneumonia in a community-based teaching hospital. Infect Control Hosp Epidemiol 1992;13:515.

139. Bartlett JG, O'Keefe P, Tally FP, et al. Bacteriology of hospital-acquired pneumonia. Arch Intern Med 1986;146:868.

140. Torres A, Puig de la Bellacasa JP, Xaubet A, et al. Diagnostic value of quantitative cultures of bronchoalveolar lavage and telescoping plugged catheters in mechanically ventilated patients with bacterial pneumonia. Am Rev Respir Dis 1989;140:306.

141. Prod'hom G, Leuenberger P, Koerfer J, et al. Nosocomial pneumonia in mechanically ventilated patients receiving antacid, rantidine, or sucralfate as prophylaxis for stress ulcer. A randomized controlled trial. Ann Intern Med 1994;120:653.

142. Rello J, Ausina V, Ricart M, et al. Impact of previous antimicrobial therapy on the etiology and outcome of ventilator-associated pneumonia. Chest 1993;104:1230.

143. Papazian L, Bregeon F, Thirion X, et al. Effect of ventilator-associated pneumonia on mortality and morbidity. Am J Respir Crit Care Med 1996;154:91.

144. Timsit J-F, Chevret S, Valcke J, et al. Mortality of nosocomial pneumonia in ventilated patients: influence of diagnostic tools. Am J Respir Crit Care Med 1996;154:116.

145. American Thoracic Society. Hospital-acquired pneumonia in adults: diagnosis, assessment of severity, initial antimicrobial therapy and preventative strategies. A consensus statements. Am Rev Resp Crit Care Med 1995;153:1711.

146. Goetz A, Yu VL. Screening for nosocomial legionellosis by culture of the water supply and targeting of high-risk patients for specialized laboratory testing. Am J Infect Control 1991;63.

147. Stout JE, Yu VL, Vickers RM, et al. Ubiquitousness of *Legionella pneumophila* in the water supply of a hospital with endemic Legionnaires' disease. N Engl J Med 1982;306:466.

148. Vickers RM, Yu VL, Hanna S, Muraca P, et al. Determinants of *Legionella pneumophila* contamination of water distribution systems: 15-hospital prospective study. Infect Control 1987;8:357.

149. Kantor HS, Poblete R, Pusateri SL. Nosocomial transmission of tuberculosis from unsuspected disease. Am J Med 1988; 84:833.

150. Catanzaro A. Nosocomial tuberculosis. Am Rev Respir Dis 1982;125:559.

151. Wenger PN, Otten J, Breeden A, et al. Control of nosocomial transmission of multidrug-resistant *Mycobacterium tuberculosis* among healthcare workers and HIV-infected patients. Lancet 1995;345:235.

152. Rhame FS. Prevention of nosocomial aspergillosis. J Hosp Infect 1991;18:466.

153. Pannuti C, Gingrich R, Pfaller MA, et al. Nosocomial pneumonia in patients having bone marrow transplant: attribute mortality and risk factors. Cancer 1992;69:2653.

154. Schwartz DN. Digest of current literature. Infect Dis Clin Pract 1996;5:538.

155. Fagon JY, Chastre J, Hance A, et al. Nosocomial pneumonia in ventilated patients: a cohort study evaluating attributable mortality and hospital stay. Am J Med 1993;94:281.

156. Silver DR, Cohen IL, Weinberg PF. Recurrent *Pseudomonas aeruginosa* pneumonia in an intensive care unit. Chest 1992;101:194.

157. Moore RD, Smith CR, Lietman PS. Association of aminoglycoside plasma levels with therapeutic outcome in gram-negative pneumonia. Am J Med 1984;77:657.

158. Torres A. Serra-Batlles J, Ros E, et al. Pulmonary aspiration of gastric contents in patients receiving mechanical ventilation: the effect of body position. Ann Intern Med 1992;116:540.

159. Driks MR, Craven DE, Celli BR, et al. Nosocomial pneumonia in intubated patients given sucralfate as compared with antacids or histamine type 2 blockers: the role of gastric colonization. N Engl J Med 1987;317:1376.

160. Valles J, Artigas A, Rello J, et al. Continuous aspiration of subglottic secretions in preventing ventilator-associated pneumonia. Ann Intern Med 1995;122:179.

161. Gastinne H, Wolff M, Delatour F, et al. A controlled trial in intensive care units of selective decontamination of the digestive tract with *nonabsorbably* antibiotics. N Engl J Med 1992;326:594.

162. Selective Decontamination of the Digestive Tract Trialists' Collaborative Group. Meta-analysis of randomised controlled trials of selective decontamination of the digestive tract. Br Med J 1993;307:525.

163. Feely TW, DuMoulin GC, Hedley-Whyte J, et al. Aerosol polymyxin and pneumonia in seriously ill patients. N Engl J Med 1975;293;471.

164. Selik RM, Chu SY, Ward JW. Trends in infectious diseases and cancers among persons dying of HIV infection in the United States from 1987 to 1992. Ann Intern Med 1995;123:933.

165. Hirschtick RE, Glassroth J, Jordan MC, et al. Bacterial pneumonia in persons infected with the human immunodeficiency virus. N Engl J Med 1995;333:845.

166. Murray JF, Garay SM, Hopewell PC, et al. Pulmonary complications of the acquired immunodeficiency syndrome: an update. Am Rev Resp Dis 1987;135:504.

167. Marston BJ, Lipman HB, Breiman RF. Surveillance for Legionnaires' disease: risk factors for mortality and morbidity. Arch Intern Med 1994;154:2417.

168. Malin AS, Gwanzura LKZ, Klein S, et al. *Pneumocystis carinii* pneumonia in Zimbabwe. Lancet 1995;346:1258.

169. Hardy WD, Feinberg J, Finkelstein DM, et al. A controlled trial of trimethoprim-sulfamethoxazole or aerosolized pentamidine for secondary prophylaxis of *Pneumocystis carinii* pneumonia in patients with acquired immunodeficiency syndrome. N Engl J Med 1992;327:1842.

170. Gallant JE, McAvinue SM, Stanton DL, et al. The impact of prophylaxis on outcome and resource utilization in *Pneumocystis carinii* pneumonia. Chest 1995;107:1018.

171. Keller DW, Breiman RF. Preventing respiratory tract infections among persons infected with human immunodeficiency virus. Clin Infect Dis 1995;21(Suppl 1):S77.

172. Selwyn PA, Hartel D, Lewis VA, et al. A prospective study of the risk of tuberculosis among intravenous drug users with human immunodeficiency virus infection. N Engl J Med 1989;320:545.

173. Bigby TD, Margolskee D, Curtis JL, et al. The usefulness of induced sputum in the diagnosis of *Pneumocystis carinii* pneumonia in patients with the acquired immunodeficiency syndrome. Am Rev Respir Dis 1986;133:515.

174. Furman AC, Jacobs J, Sepkowitz KA. Lung abscess in patients with AIDS. Clin Infect Dis 1996;22:81.

175. Bartlett JG, Gorbach SL. The triple threat of aspiration pneumonia. Chest 1975;68:560.

176. Matthay MA, Rosen GD. Acid aspiration induced lung injury. Am J Resp Crit Care Med 1996;154:277.

177. Mendelson CL. The aspiration of stomach contents into the lungs during obstetric anesthesia. Am J Obstet Gynecol 1946;52:191.

178. Bynum LJ, Pierce AK. Pulmonary aspiration of gastric contents. Am Rev Respir Dis 1976;114:1129.

179. Cameron JL, Mitchell WH, Zuidema GD. Aspiration pneumonia. Arch Surg 1973;106:49.

180. Wolfe JE, Bone RC, Ruth WE. Effects of corticosteroids in the treatment of patients with gastric aspiration. Am J Med 1977;63:719.

181. Hamelburg WV, Bosomworth PP. Aspiration pneumonitis. Springfield, IL: Charles C Thomas, 1968.

182. Bartlett JG. Anaerobic bacterial pneumonitis. Am Rev Respir Dis 1979;119:19.

183. Levison ME, Mangura CT, Lorber B, et al. Clindamycin compared with penicillin for the treatment of anaerobic lung abscess. Ann Intern Med 1983;98:466.

184. Gudiol F, Manresa F, Pallares R, et al. Clindamycin vs. penicillin for anaerobic lung infections: high rate of penicillin failures associated with penicillin-resistant *Bacteroides melaninogenicus*. Arch Intern Med 1990;150:2525.

185. Germaud P, Poirier J, Jacqueme P, et al. Monotherapy using amoxicillin/clavulanic acid as treatment of first choice in community-acquired lung abscess. Apropos of 57 cases. Rev Pneumol Clin 1993;49:137.

186. Bartlett JG. Bacterial infections of the pleural space. Semin Respir Infect 1988;3:308.

187. Light RW. Pleural disease. Baltimore: Williams & Wilkins, 1995.

188. Heffron R. Pneumonia. Cambridge, MA: Harvard University Press, 1939;566–585.

189. Bartlett JG. Empyema. In: Gorbach SL, Bartlett JG, Blacklow NR, eds. Infectious Diseases. Philadelphia: WB Saunders, in press.

190. Deschamps C, Allen MS, Trastek VA, et al. Empyema following pulmonary resection. Chest Surg Clin N Am 1994;4:583.

191. Bartlett JG, Gorbach SL, Thadepalli H, et al. Bacteriology of empyema. Lancet 1974;1:338.

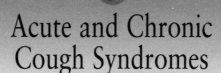

Acute and Chronic Cough Syndromes

John G. Bartlett

Bronchitis

Snapshot Summary

Acute bronchitis

Clinical features: Acute upper respiratory infection (URI) associated with a cough producing purulent sputum.

Etiology

Common: viral infection

Uncommon but treatable with antimicrobials: *Mycoplasma pneumoniae*, *Chlamydia pneumoniae*, pertussis, influenza.

Diagnostic studies: usually none

Treatment: symptomatic

Antibiotics are *not* indicated

Exacerbations of chronic bronchitis

Clinical features: Chronic bronchitis with an increase in cough, dyspnea, and/or sputum purulence.

Etiology: Viral URI, environmental irritant, subclinical asthma. The role of bacterial infection is unclear despite extensive and often elegant studies in thousands of patients, including sputum cultures, quantitative sputum bacteriology, transtracheal aspirations, and sputum cytologic analysis. Meta-analysis shows a slight advantage with antibiotics directed against *Hemophilus influenzae* and *Streptococcus pneumoniae.*

Diagnostic tests: usually none; sputum bacteriology is usually not helpful.

Treatment: respiratory support

Antibiotics: "traditional agents," such as doxycycline, amoxicillin, TMP-SMX.

Preferred agents for *H. influenzae* and *S. pneumoniae:* azithromycin, levofloxacin, sparfloxacin, cefpodoxime, cefuroxime, cefprozil.

Chronic cough syndromes (not caused by chronic bronchitis)

Condition	%	History/PE	Test
Post-nasal drip syndrome	40-50%	Sensation of post-nasal drainage; purulent secretions nose	CT scan sinuses
Asthma	20-25%	Wheezing	Pulmonary function test
Gastro-esophageal reflux	20-25%	Heartburn and "waterbrash"	Barium esophagography

Miscellaneous causes: Bronchiectasis, adrenal cortical extract (ACE) inhibitor, interstitial pulmonary fibrosis.

Bronchitis is one of the most common conditions encountered in clinical practice. In general, there are two main categories: acute bronchitis and exacerbations of chronic bronchitis. Related syndromes based on shared clinical features are the postnasal drip syndrome subclinical asthma, gastrointestinal reflux, sinusitis and a miscellany of relatively rare conditions. Infection is only one of the multiple causes of bronchitis. Bronchitis, which has been known throughout the history of medicine, is clearly more common since the Industrial Revolution and the widespread use of cigarettes. This chapter deals with the clinical features of acute and chronic bronchitis and provides guidelines for medical management. Also included is a discussion of other causes of acute and chronic cough syndromes.

Acute Bronchitis

DEFINITION

Acute bronchitis is an isolated event characterized by inflammation of the bronchi and clinically expressed with a cough that is usually accompanied by sputum production. There may be associated fever and constitutional complaints. The major considerations in differential diagnosis are pneumonia and upper airway conditions such as sinusitis or allergic rhinitis with bronchial drainage. Pneumonia can usually be distinguished with a chest radiograph showing the absence of a new pulmonary infiltrate. Upper airway conditions can be detected by the symptom complex, although bronchitis is often concurrent with an upper airway infection. A cough is common with most upper respiratory tract viral infections, including the usual agents of the common cold such as rhinovirus, influenza, parainfluenza, coronavirus, and respiratory syncytial virus (RSV).

ETIOLOGY

Infectious causes of acute bronchitis are primarily viral; they include influenza A and B, parainfluenza, rhinovirus, coronavirus, and RSV (Table 2.1). Potentially treatable agents of acute bronchitis in the immunocompetent host are infections caused by *Mycoplasma pneumoniae*, *Chlamydia pneumoniae*, and *Bordetella pertussis*. There is often suspicion of acute bacterial bronchitis involving

Table 2.1
Acute Bronchitis: Infectious Agents and Treatment

Agent	Treatment
VIRAL	
Influenza A	Amantadine or rimantadine
Influenza B	—
Parainfluenza	—
Coronavirus	—
Respiratory syncytial virus	—
Rhinovirus	—
BACTERIA AND BACTERIALIKE	
Mycoplasma pneumoniae	Doxycycline or macrolide[a]
Chlamydia pneumoniae	Doxycycline or macrolide[a]
Bordetella pertussis	Erythromycin

[a]Macrolide, erythromycin, azithromycin, clarithromycin.

common respiratory tract pathogens such as *S. pneumoniae, H. influenzae, S. aureus,* and *Moraxella catarrhalis;* nevertheless, no evidence of "bacterial bronchitis" is found except possibly in neonates, patients with airway violations (tracheostomy or endotracheal intubation), or in immunosuppressed hosts. Following is a discussion of the major causes of bronchitis symptoms that are treatable and epidemiologically important.

Mycoplasma pneumoniae. The epidemiology of *M. pneumoniae* shows high rates at 4- to 5-year cycles. This common infection in young adults has clinical features that include pharyngitis, fever, constitutional symptoms, and extrapulmonary complications (4,5). The disease course is usually self-limited with recovery in 1–2 weeks, but some cases are relatively chronic and may persist with typical symptoms, including a cough, for up to 4–6 weeks. The cough is often accompanied mucoid sputum production that shows mononuclear cells and sparse organisms on Gram stain.

The diagnosis may be established by culture of *M. pneumoniae* from pharyngeal washings, acute and convalescent sera showing a fourfold rise in titer, an elevated serum IgM titer (6), or antigen detection with polymerase chain reaction (PCR) (7). Many laboratories do not offer any of these tests. A cold agglutinin titer of 1:64 or greater is highly suggestive. The titer tends to correlate with disease severity. None of these diagnostic studies are realistic for most patients owing to cost, lack of availability, or non-specificity.

The preferred treatment is doxycycline or a macrolide (8). Tetracyclines should be avoided in pregnant women and in children aged younger than 17 years. Erythromycin is equally effective, but it is poorly tolerated by many patients. Other drugs that are active in vitro are azithromycin, clarithromycin, and fluoroquinolones (ofloxacin, levofloxacin, sparfloxacin, ciprofloxacin) (8,9). With treatment, most patients have a clinical response: fever resolves within 1–2 days and the cough in 2–3 days. Treatment should be continued 3 weeks to prevent relapses. Curiously, the pathogen is not eliminated with treatment so that *M. pneumoniae* may still be transmitted to close contacts (10).

Chlamydia pneumoniae. This is a relatively newly recognized "bacterialike agent" that was initially called the "TWAR agent" as a method to combine the original appellations: the "Taiwan agent" and the "acute respiratory agent" (11).

Clinical features of *C. pneumoniae* often include pharyngitis, laryngitis, and bronchitis. Common features are hoarseness, low-grade fever, and a persistent cough. Pneumonitis may be present (11) and some adults or children have exacerbation of asthma (12). As with *M. pneumoniae,* the most susceptible patients appear to be young adults aged between 5 and 20 years; nevertheless, this pathogen can afflict older adults as well. Serologic surveys suggest that about 50% of adults have had previous infections, but conclusions are limited by concerns about the specificity of the serologic test (13). The most characteristic feature of *C. pneumoniae* bronchitis is the persistent, hacking cough that may or may not produce mucoid sputum. Microscopic examination of sputum shows mononuclear cells and sparse bacteria. The disease usually lasts 2–3 weeks without treatment, but may persist for several weeks (14).

Chlamydia pneumoniae is a relatively new respiratory tract pathogen and diagnostic studies are poorly defined. Most authorities feel the most definitive test is a serologic response (preferably the microimmunofluorescent assay or MIF) combined with evidence of the pathogen by culture that requires the tissue culture technique or polymerase chain reaction (PCR) (15,16). As noted, serologic tests reported in most studies are of concern owing to their nonspecificity. For practical purposes, most physicians do not have access to laboratories that have the diagnostic resources to identify *C. pneumoniae.*

Treatment consists of drugs that are effective in vitro including tetracyclines, macrolides (erythromycin, clarithromycin, azithromycin), and fluoroquinolones (ofloxacin, levofloxacin, sparfloxacin, ciprofloxacin) (17). Most patients respond with resolution of symptoms within 3–5 days. Treatment is continued 10–14 days.

Pertussis. Pertussis is a disease that caused substantial morbidity and mortality before the mid-1940s when the vaccine was introduced. Since then, the number of cases has declined in the United States from a peak of 260,000 in 1934 to a historic low of 1010 cases in 1976 (18).

The epidemiology since the early 1980s shows periodic increases in the reported cases of pertussis in the United States and this presumably applies to other countries that have widespread use of pertussis vaccine (19). Current case rates in the United States are 1.5–3.0 per 100,000 population. Pertussis is traditionally viewed as primarily a disease of children, but about 30% of cases are reported in persons more than 10 years of age. A recent study of 153 adults evaluated in Kaiser, San Francisco for chronic cough persisting 2 or more weeks showed 12% had evidence of pertussis (20). Of particular interest was the observation that this diagnosis was not specifically suspected by the physician in any of these patients.

To prevent pertussis, the current immunization recommendation is three doses of DTP (diphtheria, tetanus, and pertussis) at ages 2 months, 4 months, 6 months, 12–18 months, and at 4–6 years. The experience with this vaccine shows it provides 64% protection against mild disease and 95% protection against severe disease (21). Patients at greatest risk are those who have not received the vaccine, primarily infants, but also some adults. Exposure is obviously necessary so that the infected infant may become the source of infection for close contacts, including family members, school mates, other persons in day care centers, and so forth.

The major clinical feature in adults is a barking cough that is often so prominent and severe that the patient has difficulty completing a sentence. Another feature is cough persistence for 3 or more weeks in 80% of adults with pertussis (22).

The diagnosis is established with a "cough plate" in which the agar plate appropriate for culture of B. pertussis is held before the patient's mouth for an aerosolized inoculation during a typical coughing bout. The alternative is a nasopharyngeal aspirate (23). PCR technology is available, but not yet in widespread use (24). The treatment of pertussis is with erythromycin as the standard drug; alternatives include ampicillin, chloramphenicol, and trimethoprim-sulfamethoxazole (25).

Influenza. Influenza is undoubtedly the most serious viral airway infection in terms of morbidity and mortality (26–30). The epidemiology is seasonal (winter months), global, and type-specific (28). Strain variations are noted each year with antigenic shifts and drifts; a shift indicates a major antigenic change and a drift implies a minor change (30). The practical implications of these differences concern antigen specificity with the extent of humoral protection dependent on prior antigenic experience from vaccination and clinical infection. Major influenza epidemics are associated with 20,000 or more deaths in the United States ascribed to influenza and pneumonia (30).

Prevention is primarily accomplished by annual vaccination, which is advocated for elderly patients, patients rendered vulnerable to consequences of influenza by associated diseases, and health care workers who could pose a risk to patients (30,31). Each year, the prediction of the predominant epidemic strain determines the vaccine advocated for susceptible hosts with the usual recommendation for administration at 1–3 months before the anticipated epidemic. In most seasons, global trends predict epidemic strain(s) that are then used to construct the annual vaccine. Primarily targeted for the vaccine are persons aged 65 years or older, residents of nursing homes, and persons with cardiopulmonary disease. Vaccine efficacy is usually 60%–70% to prevent transmission; in the elderly, the protection is less effective, but efficacy in preventing mortality is usually 70%–80% (29). In general, influenza A is more severe and shows greater antigenic heterogeneity compared with influenza B. H_3N_2 strains are associated with the highest mortality rates (30).

Clinical features of influenza include upper respiratory complaints that are usually accompanied by bronchitis with the production of purulent sputum. Constitutional symptoms, such as fever, fatigue, and malaise, may be profound. The most susceptible to severe consequences are found in patients in the age extremes (infants and elderly patients), infants due to antigenic naivete and the elderly because of multiple confounding associated diseases. More than 90% of deaths ascribed to influenza and its complications are in elderly patients, especially occupants of chronic care facilities because of clustering of highly vulnerable patients. Multiple complications are associated with influenza (Table 2.2), but the most common are pulmonary complications in patients who are elderly or have pre-existing pulmonary or cardiovascular disease.

The diagnosis is established by viral culture or fluorescent stain of respiratory secretions or by demonstration of seroconversion with acute and convalescent sera. Culture is important for epidemiologic tracking of strains so that the epidemic strain can be typed to document the presence of an influenza epidemic and to characterize the strain, which is done for public health purposes. For the individual patient, the diagnosis is usually based on the recognition of typical clinical symptoms with an exposure history in a location associated with an influenza epidemic.

Treatment using amantadine or rimantadine is available for patients with infections involving influenza A. These drugs are active only against influenza A so that the predominant epidemiologic strain is important to know when considering these drugs. Clinical benefit is documented only if these drugs are given within 48 hours of the onset of symptoms (32). Therapeutic trials have shown that these drugs are somewhat more effective than aspirin or similar anti-inflammatory agents (33). In vitro resistance to both drugs has been documented and use of amantadine or rimantadine has been associated with transmission of strains of influenza A within households that are resistant (34). The major concern with influenza is the possibility of complications, which are summarized in Table 2.2. Many

Table 2.2
Complications of Influenza

Complication	Comment
PULMONARY	
Primary influenza pneumonia (38)	Risk factors: Cardiovascular disease and pregnancy
	Uncommon since 1957–1958 epidemic
	Clinical feature: Bilateral infiltrates, leukocytosis, high mortality rate
	Autopsies show tracheitis, bronchitis, hemorrhagic pneumonia with few inflammatory cells
Bacterial superinfection (39,40)	Risk factors: Pulmonary disease and age >65 yrs
	Clinical features: Classic influenza → improvement → recurrent fever with cough and purulent sputum
	Radiograph: unilateral infiltrate, leukocytosis Agents: *Streptococcus pneumoniae* (most common), *Staphylococcus aureus* (most lethal); others: *H. influenzae, Neisseria meningitidis, S. pyogenes*
Mixed pattern	Combination of above
Chronic lung disease: Exacerbation of bronchitis	Common cause of exacerbation of chronic bronchitis
Asthma	May cause status asthmaticus
NON PULMONARY	
Myositis (41,42)	Tender leg muscles with elevated creatinine phosphokinase
Cardiac (43,44)	Myocarditis or pericarditis
Toxic shock syndrome (45)	Ascribed to superinfection by *S. aureus* or *S. pyogenes*
Neurologic complications (46–48)	Guillain-Barré syndrome, encephalitis, transverse myelitis
Reye's syndrome (49)	Hepatic and central nervous complication in children aged 2–16 yrs
	Primarily due to influenza B

patients have prolonged periods in which pulmonary function is reduced despite lack of X-ray evidence of pneumonia (35,36).

The major recognized complications are pulmonary involvement with primary influenza pneumonia or a bacterial superinfection (37). The classic description of the latter is influenza that is clinically improving followed by symptom recurrence at 7–10 days after the original onset of symptoms. This complication is most common in the elderly, especially persons in nursing homes, and is easily detected with a chest radiograph showing an infiltrate; the absence of an infiltrate virtually excludes bacterial superinfection of the lung. The major superinfecting pathogens are *S. pneumoniae,* which is the most common, and *S. aureus,* which causes the most severe disease. Other superinfecting pathogens that are less common are *H. influenzae, Neisseria meningitidis,* and group A beta-hemolytic streptococcus. Influenza with superinfection by *S. aureus* or group A streptococcus may be complicated by toxic shock syndrome. This may account for the rare cases of devastating disease in young adults. Other extrapulmonary complications include myositis (41,42), pericarditis (43), myocarditis (44), toxic shock syndrome (45), Guillian-Barré syndrome (46), encephalitis (47,48), and, in pediatric patients, Reye's syndrome (49).

DIAGNOSIS

Most previously healthy adults with typical symptoms of bronchitis do not require diagnostic evaluation other than reassurance. Symptoms suggesting that medical intervention might be appropriate include fever, profound constitutional symptoms, dyspnea, rigors, or pleurisy. The medical evaluation should be driven by symptoms, age, associated diseases, and epidemiologic patterns. Patients with a cough that is incapacitating or persists for more than 2 weeks often have something other than a common viral infection; the diagnostic possibilities include treatable pathogens such as *M. pneumoniae, C. pneumoniae,* and *B. pertussis.* Physical examination of these patients is usually focused on both the upper and lower respiratory tracts. It is important to acknowledge that sinusitis and allergic rhinitis may present with symptoms of bronchitis, which requires attention to the upper respiratory tract evaluation. In general, the most definitive test is a radio-graph or computed tomography (CT) scan of sinuses, but for cost and practical reasons, the most realistic evaluation consists of bedside tests, including a good history, palpation over frontal and maxillary sinuses, nasal examination, and transillumination (50). Patients with viral infections often have mucous membrane erythema of the upper airways, including nasal passages and pharynx. Exudative pharyngitis is unusual with *M. pneumoniae* or *C. pneumoniae.*

Pulmonary parenchyma involvement with pneumonia can be definitively detected only with a good auscultatory examination showing fine crackles (rales) and a pulmonary infiltrate on a chest radiograph. The chest radiograph is regarded as the most definitive test but repeating the radiograph in 24 or more hours may be necessary if the patient is seen early in the disease course. Critical factors in evaluation of possible treatable agents include symptom duration, cough characteristics, severe constitutional symptoms, dyspnea, and hypoxemia. Documented fever or persistence of a cough for more than 2 weeks usually merits evaluation with a chest radiograph as a minimal diagnostic evaluation. Most patients will simply have an acute syndrome characterized by upper respiratory symptoms (nasal discharge, sore throat, laryngitis) and an acute cough that may be productive of purulent sputum. Such patients do not require any diagnostic or therapeutic intervention other than reassurance and an appropriate message regarding contagion. Pertussis must be excluded in patients with an incapacitating cough that persists longer than 2 weeks (Table 2.3).

Table 2.3
Clinical Features of 19 Adult Patients with Pertussis[a]

Age	
(mean)	42 yrs
(range)	24–78 yrs
Duration of cough	
(mean)	8 wks
(range)	2–14 wks
Immunization history	
Childhood	9
No history	10
Signs and symptoms	
Paroxysmal cough	16
Fever	5
Sputum production	15

[a]Adapted from: Nennig ME, Shinefield HR, Edwards KM, et al. Prevalence and incidence of adult pertussis in an urban population. JAMA 1996;275:1672. Diagnosis was based on enzyme-linked immunosorbent assay of IgG antibodies to pertussis toxin.

Microbiology. For individual patient management, diagnostic studies to detect causative agents, as reviewed above, are seldom indicated. In epidemics it may be important to identify selected epidemiologically important pathogens such as pertussis, influenza, and possibly *M. pneumoniae*. Even when antibiotics are prescribed, an etiologic diagnosis is usually not established because the major treatable agents (influenza A, *C. pneumoniae*, and *M. pneumoniae*) are not detected by most laboratories. A possible exception is *B. pertussis*.

TREATMENT

Most patients with acute bronchitis require no specific treatment and only "nonspecific agents" to reduce constitutional complaints using anti-inflammatory agents and possibly cough suppressants. For patients with a severe cough, prolonged cough, or infections associated with constitutional symptoms including fever, most physicians will prescribe antibiotics (51) despite the lack of a confirmed benefit (52,53). Several trials have demonstrated that oral betalactam drugs with activity versus *S. pneumoniae*, *H. influenzae*, and *M. catarrhalis* effectively eliminate the suspected pathogen in such cases (51–58). The problem is that these are not quality studies because of the lack of placebo-control format, small sample size, and poor assessment of compliance (54). Furthermore, likely treatable pathogens include agents that are often resistant to betalactam drugs such as penicillin-resistant *S. pneumoniae*, *H. influenzae*, *M. pneumoniae*, *C. pneumoniae*, and influenza. During an influenza epidemic, the patient who has typical symptoms usually receives only symptomatic treatment, although rimantadine and amantadine are potentially useful in this setting. For patients more than 55 years of age with frequent cough and systemic complaints, one option is doxycycline, 100 mg twice daily for 5–10 days (52). Advantages include activity against most bacterial pathogens and atypical pathogens, low price, good tolerance, and modest efficacy in at least one recent controlled study (52), although the latter point is debated (53). The major alternatives are macrolides or fluoroquinolones based on activity in vitro against likely pathogens. For pertussis, the drug of choice is erythromycin.

Exacerbations of Chronic Bronchitis

DEFINITION

Chronic bronchitis is characterized by cough and sputum production over an extended period. Arbitrarily, the standard definition is a productive cough and sputum production for 3 months per year for at least 2 years that is not caused by other conditions such as tuberculosis or bronchiectasis. Chronic bronchitis and emphysema are components of chronic obstructive pulmonary disease (COPD) (59), which represents a heterogeneous group of clinical conditions and collectively represents the fifth leading cause of death in the United States. Acute exacerbations of chronic bronchitis are defined as a worsening of clinical symptoms with increased cough, increased sputum production, and increased dyspnea. Some cases are accompanied by fever and some patients have symptoms consistent with asthma, leading to the term "asthmatic bronchitis" (60,61). Hemoptysis may also be seen during acute exacerbations; chronic bronchitis is the most common cause of hemoptysis in developed countries.

ETIOLOGY

The most common cause of chronic bronchitis and COPD is smoking (61,62). Air pollution and occupational exposure are less common. "Industrial bronchitis" is a term used for bronchitis resulting from occupational exposure to dust, gas, or fumes (63,64). A genetic basis is noted with severe alpha-1 globulin deficiency, cystic fibrosis, immunoglobulin deficiencies (congenital or acquired), and "primary ciliary dyskinesia." Some patients with asthma have hypersecretion of mucus leading to symptoms of both chronic bronchitis and asthma (60,61).

Exacerbations may occur from any of the following: smoking, air pollution, allergens, occupational exposure, or preclinical and subclinical asthma. Infection is thought to be an important cause, but this has been difficult to prove based on microbiology studies or with placebo-controlled trials of antibiotic treatment. The organisms most commonly implicated are viral agents that often cause upper respiratory tract infections and two major bacterial species: *S. pneumoniae* and *H. influenzae*. Most exacerbations ascribed to infection are thought to represent viral infections of the upper airways. Chronic bronchitis is one of the most extensively and best studied conditions in medicine, but conclusions regarding the role of infections as a cause of acute exacerbations are inconclusive. Infections do not appear to promote the basic disease process with progressive deterioration in pulmonary function (62). The following conclusions can be made on the basis of available data:

1. Viral infections: The frequency of viral respiratory tract infection in association with acute exacerbations of chronic bronchitis ranges from 7% to 64% (65–69). Perhaps the best of the studies is by Gump, et al. (66) who found viral infections in 32% of patients during exacerbations compared with 1% during remissions. The viruses most commonly found by viral culture or serology are influenza A or B, parainfluenza virus, coronavirus, and rhinovirus (65–71).

2. Sputum cytology: The role of bacterial infection in exacerbations of chronic bronchitis and in progression of disease has been examined by sequential cultures, response rates to antibiotics in controlled clinical trials, and sputum cytology. Sputum cytology is based on quantitative assessment of expectorated secretions collected sequentially over a period of years, both during exacerbations and during periods of relative quiescence (72,73). Results indicate large concentrations of inflammatory cells including polymorphonuclear cells throughout the course of chronic bronchitis without notable changes during exacerbations. Thus, the perception of increased purulence cannot be necessarily confirmed by the concentration of leukocytes or the distribution of cells in expectorated secretions. Biopsies of bronchi in chronic bronchitis show increased mucosal and mural inflammation with increased numbers of macrophages and both CD4 and CD8 lymphocytes (74–76).

3. Cultures: Multiple studies have shown that cultures of expectorated secretions in patients with chronic

bronchitis give a high yield of potential respiratory
tract pathogens during both exacerbations and remissions. Arguably, the most comprehensive studies were
done by Gump, et al. (66) who followed 25 patients
with chronic bronchitis with evaluations at 2-week in-
tervals for 4 years (Table 2.4). Cultures of sputum
were obtained at each visit. This work showed comparable rates of recovery of *S. pneumoniae, H. influen-*

Table 2.4
Microbiologic Studies During Exacerbations and Remissions of Chronic Bronchitis[a]

	Exacerbations		Remissions	
	No.	Positive	No.	Positive
Viral cultures positive	116	38 (32%)	4034	35 (0.9%)
Bacterial cultures				
Staphylococcus pneumoniae	86	32 (37%)	1267	419 (33%)
Hemophilus influenzae	86	49 (57%)	1267	759 (60%)
Staphylococcus aureus	86	12 (14%)	1267	232 (18%)
Candida species	86	25 (29%)	1267	232 (18%)
Gram-negative bacilli	86	25 (29%)	1267	598 (47%)
Quantitative cultures				
S. pneumoniae $\geq 10^6$	83	21 (25%)	1240	228 (18%)

[a]Adapted from: Gump DW, Phillips CA, Forsyth BR, et al. Role of
infection in chronic bronchitis. Am Rev Respir Dis 1976;113:465.
Based on a prospective longitudinal study of 25 patients with
chronic bronchitis followed with clinic evaluations at 2-week inter-
vals for 4 years. There were 116 exacerbations observed with a total
of 4150 patient weeks.

zae, and other potential pathogens during both exacerbations and remissions; the mean counts of *S. pneumoniae* were generally 10^7/mL. The yield of *S. pneumoniae* in this study was 37% in exacerbations and 33% in remissions. Others report a yield of 15%–50% (77–79). The same applies to *H. influenzae,* except the yield is higher (79,80). Nearly all strains of *H. influenzae* are nontypable (79). Transtracheal aspirates on many patients with COPD and chronic bronchitis show high rates of lower airway colonization by bacteria that is not seen in healthy controls; the dominant organisms are *S. pneumoniae, H. influenzae,* and nonpathogens such as alpha-hemolytic streptococci and *H. parainfluenzae* (77,80,81). These studies collectively show that patients with chronic bronchitis have high rates of colonization with *S. pneumoniae* and *H. influenzae,* and this colonization extends to the tracheobronchial tract below the level of the larynx. This work also shows that acute exacerbations cannot be distinguished from quiescent periods in patients with chronic bronchitis by bacterial culture or even by quantitative culture of respiratory secretions.

4. Antibiotic trials: The only guidelines on management of exacerbations of bronchitis from the American Thoracic Society were published in 1987 (62). These state: "Although antibiotics have been used extensively for years to treat acute exacerbations of chronic bronchitis, as well as for prophylaxis in stable bronchitis, their value for either purpose has not been established." Many would argue that this conclusion applies 10 years later. A problem is that there are multiple studies of antibiotic treatment of chronic bronchitis exacerbations, but relatively few had an appropriate study format for scientific validity (82–93). Among those considered adequate trials, the antibiotics tested comprises a relatively short list:

amoxicillin, tetracyclines, trimethoprim-sulfamethoxazole, or chloramphenicol. One of the largest and best studies in recent years was a double-blind placebo-controlled trial of 173 patients with 362 exacerbations by Anthonisen, et al. (85), who showed accelerated clinical recovery in 68% of antibiotic recipients compared with 55% of the placebo group. This difference was statistically significant; there was also a modest, but statistically significant improvement in peak flow rates. Findings are summarized in Table 2.5. Other studies show similar results. Saint, et al. recently provided a meta-analysis of published trials that addresses the issue of antibiotic treatment for exacerbations of chronic pulmonary disease (84). A MEDLINE search for 1955 to 1994 showed only 9 of 214 reports satisfied the selection criteria for randomized trials with antibiotic treatment versus placebo (Table 2.6). Antibiotics evaluated were limited: tetracyclines, chloramphenicol, ampicillin, and TMP-SMX.

Table 2.5
Controlled Trial of Antibiotic Treatment of Exacerbations of Chronic Bronchitis[a]

		Treatment Success	
	No.	Placebo	Antibiotic
Type of exacerbation			
Increased dyspnea, sputum, *and* sputum purulence	137	31/69 (43%)	44/68 (63%)
Two of the above three	147	45/73 (60%)	54/74 (76%)
One of the above three	67	23/33 (70%)	26/34 (74%)

[a]Adapted from: Anthonisen NR, Manfreda J, Warren CPW, et al. Antibiotic therapy in exacerbations of chronic obstructive pulmonary disease. Ann Intern Med 1987;106:196.

Table 2.6

Antibiotics for Exacerbations of Chronic Obstructive Pulmonary Disease: Meta-Analysis[a]

Study	No.	Setting	Antibiotic	Outcome	Result[b]
Elmes, et al. 1957 (86)	113	OPD	Tetracycline	Days of illness	Benefit NS
Berry, et al. 1960 (90)	33	OPD	Tetracycline	Symptom score	Benefit Sig
Fear and Edwards 1962 (91)	119	OPD	Tetracycline	Symptom score	Benefit NS
Elmes, et al. 1965 (87)	56	Hosp pts	Ampicillin	PEFR	Benefit NS
Peterson, et al. 1967 (92)	19	Hosp pts	Chloramphenicol	PEFR	No benefit NS
Pines, et al. 1968 (89)	149	Hosp pts	Tetracycline	Symptom score PEFR	Benefit Sig
Nicotra, et al. 1982 (88)	40	Hosp pts	Tetracycline	Days of illness PEFR	Benefit NS
Anthonisen 1987 (85)	310	OPD	TMP-SMX, amoxicillin, or doxycycline	Days of illness PEFR	Benefit Sig
Jurgensen 1992 (93)	262	OPD	Amoxicillin	Symptom score PEFR	No benefit NS

[a]Data from: Saint S, Bent S, Vittinghoff E, et al. Antibiotics in chronic obstructive pulmonary exacerbations: a meta-analysis. JAMA 1995;273:957.
[b]Results show benefit favoring antibiotic treatment. Individual studies evaluated for significance of difference for outcome measured. NS, not statistically significant; Sig, statistically significant. The overall results showed a small but statistically significant benefit with antibiotic treatment.
OPD, outpatients; Hosp pts, hospitalized patients; PEFR, Peak expiratory flow rates.

Outcomes evaluated were also diverse: days of illness, symptom score, physician evaluation, or peak expiratory flow rate (PEFR). Results were variable, but seven of the nine studies showed a benefit with treatment and the overall result showed a small, but statistically significant, improvement. Analysis of the six studies that measured PEFR showed an improvement of 10.75 L/min, a very modest improvement favoring antibiotic treatment.

DIAGNOSIS

Patients with exacerbations of bronchitis need to be evaluated for the severity of symptoms to determine the need for hospitalization, supportive care, and antibiotic treatment. Patients with fever or crackles should usually have a chest radiograph to evaluate for pneumonitis. The utility of Gram stain and culture of expectorated secretions is debated. Most advise not to bother.

TREATMENT

Treatment consists of supportive care and antibiotics directed against *S. pneumoniae* and *H. influenzae*. As noted, the role of bacteria is often unclear and most authorities recommend antibiotics only in patients with severe exacerbations or in those associated with fever. Standard treatment usually consists of a 10- to 14-day course of amoxicillin, doxycycline, or trimethoprim-sulfamethoxazole. These are the drugs that have been used most extensively in therapeutic trials showing benefit (84). Many other drugs are possibly more logical choices based on in vitro sensitivity tests of the two major pathogens including azithromycin, cefpodoxime, cefprozil, cefuroxime, ofloxacin, levofloxacin, and sparfloxacin. None of these have proved superior to the standard drugs in adequately controlled comparative trials, but they may be preferred owing to enhanced activity against anticipated pathogens.

PREVENTION

Patients with chronic bronchitis and COPD should receive influenza vaccine annually and pneumococcal vaccine once with possible readministration at 6 years. The utility of influenza vaccine is well established for reducing both the rate and the severity of symptoms with influenza (95). With pneumococcal vaccine, no evidence exists for a reduction in the frequency or severity of exacerbations in patients with chronic bronchitis (96,97). The recommendation is made with the assumption that it will reduce the frequency of pneumococcal pneumonia. Some physicians advocate prophylactic antibiotics for patients with severe exacerbations, especially when this can be confined to specific months associated with high risk for multiple exacerbations (98–100). The usual recommendation is one of the three antibiotics noted previously: amoxicillin, doxycycline, or trimethoprim-sulfamethoxazole. These may be given continuously or on a rotational basis. Again, there may be interest in using newer agents with enhanced activity versus *S. pneumoniae* and *H. influenzae*. Problems with this tactic are the lack of demonstrable benefit in terms of documented clinical efficacy or cost-effectiveness, and the potential hazards of side effects, cost, and resistance.

Acute and Chronic Cough: Other Causes

CHRONIC COUGH

A cough is defined as chronic when it persists for 3 weeks. Chronic bronchitis from smoking or environmental irritants is the most common cause. For nonsmoking patients, the most common cause is the postnasal drip syndrome followed by asthma and gastroesophageal reflux (Table 2.7). The diagnostic evaluation should include a history, physical examination, and chest radiograph. Patients who smoke and those exposed to environmental

Table 2.7

Differential Diagnosis of Chronic Cough[a]

Condition	Frequency	Features
Postnasal drip syndrome	40%–50%	Hx: Sensation of secretion passage down throat, nasal discharge, frequent need to clear throat PE: Mucoid or mucopurulent secretion and/or cobblestone changes in nasopharynx or oropharynx Test: Rule out sinusitis—CT or sinuses
Asthma	20%–25%	Hx: Episodic wheezing PE: Wheezing Test: Pulmonary function testing shows reversible airway obstruction (FEV$_1$ increased ≥15% from baseline after albuterol or positive methacholine inhalation)
Gastroesophageal reflux	20%–25%	Hx: Heartburn and sour taste in mouth ≥3 weeks Test: Barium esophagography or esophageal pH monitoring
Bronchiectasis	4%	Hx: Purulent sputum production Test: Radiograph shows increased size or loss of definition of marking in segmented regions, cystic spaces, honeycombing, compensatory hyperinflation, or high resolution CT shows bronchiectasis
ACE inhibitor		Hx: Receiving ACE inhibitor
Interstitial pulmonary fibrosis		Test: Pulmonary function tests show restrictive pattern; radiograph shows interstitial changes and/or biopsy shows this diagnosis

[a]Adapted from:. Am Rev Respir Dis 1990;141:642 and Mello CJ, Irwin RS, Curley FJ. Predictive values of character, timing, and complications of chronic cough in diagnosing its cause. Arch Intern Med 1996;156:997.
ACE, adrenal cortex extract; CT, computed tomography; FEV$_1$, forced expiratory volume in 1 second; Hx, history; PE, physical examination.

irritants should eliminate these obvious causes as a therapeutic trial. If the history and physical findings suggest the postnasal drip syndrome, the following diagnostic studies are indicated: radiographs or CT scan of sinuses and an allergy evaluation. Other tests to consider in case of negative evaluation through this stage are spirometry before and after a bronchodilator to exclude asthma and then studies for gastroesophageal reflux (barium swallow, esophageal pH monitoring).

ACUTE COUGH

Acute cough is most frequently caused by the common cold. The usual symptoms are nasal discharge, nasal obstruction, throat clearing, and cough. This is, by definition, self-limited. Studies of patients with the common cold indicate the cough will have disappeared in 74% by day 14 (1).

POSTNASAL DRIP SYNDROME

Definition. The "postnasal drip syndrome" is an unscientific term used to signify a number of common clinical problems caused by conditions of the upper respiratory tract characterized by postnasal drip. It is included in this discussion because a cough is a common clinical feature, and this is often mistaken as bronchitis.

Clinical features. Postnasal drip syndrome should be considered in patients who describe the sensation of a postnasal drainage that often results in a cough or in a need to clear the throat. Physical examination of the upper airways usually shows mucoid or mucopurulent secretions.

Etiology. The usual causes include the common cold, allergic rhinitis, vasomotor rhinitis, postinfectious rhinitis, sinusitis, drug-induced conditions (primarily ACE inhibitors), and environmental irritants (94).

Table 2.8
Causes and Treatment of Postnasal Drip Syndrome

Cause	Treatment
Allergic rhinitis	Intranasal beclomethasone ± antihistamine/ decongestant
	Avoid precipitating factor
Vasomotor rhinitis	Intranasal beclomethasone ± antihistamine/ decongestant
	Intranasal ipratropium bromide
Environmental irritant	Intranasal beclomethasone ± antihistamine/ decongestant
	Avoid irritant if feasible
Postinfectious rhinitis	Intranasal beclomethasone ± antihistamine/ decongestant
Sinusitis	Antibiotic decongestant nasal spray (oxymetazoline HCl) and + dexbrompheniramine maleate + d-isoephedrine

Treatment. Treatment for the postnasal drip syndrome is summarized in Table 2.8 and consists primarily of intranasal beclomethasone vipropionate sometimes accompanied by an antihistamine/decongestant. Irritants responsible should obviously be avoided. Sinusitis may require antibiotic treatment and/or a decongestant nasal spray.

References

1. Dingle JH, Badger GF, Jordon WS Jr. Illness in the home: a study of 25,000 illnesses in a group of Cleveland families. Cleveland: The Press of Western Reserve University, 1964:68.
2. Gwaltney JM Jr: Rhinoviruses. In: Evans AS, ed. Viral infections of humans: epidemiology and control, 3rd ed. New York: Plenum, 1989:593.

3. Tyrrell DAJ. Common colds and related diseases. Baltimore: Williams & Wilkins, 1965.

4. Foy HM, Kenny GE, McMahan R, et al. *Mycoplasma pneumoniae* pneumonia in an urban area. JAMA 1970;214:1966.

5. Denny FW, Clyde WA, Glenzen WP. *Mycoplasma pneumoniae* disease. Clinical spectrum, pathophysiology, epidemiology and control. J Infect Dis 1971;123:74.

6. Uldum SA, Jensen JS, Sondergard-Anderson J, et al. Enzyme immunoassay for detection of immunoglobulin M (IgM) and IgG antibodies to *Mycoplasma pneumoniae*. J Clin Microbiol 1992;30:1198.

7. Dular R, Kajioka R, Kasatiya S. Comparison of Gen-Probe commercial kit and culture technique for the diagnosis of *Mycoplasma pneumoniae* infection. J Clin Microbiol 1988; 26:1068.

8. Rylander M, Hallander HO. In vitro comparison of the activity of doxycycline, tetracycline, erythromycin and a new macrolide, CP 62993, against Mycoplasma pneumoniae, *Mycoplasma hominis* and *Ureaplasma urealyticum*. Scand J Infect Dis 1988;53(Suppl):12.

9. Cassell GH, Waites KB, Pate MS, et al. Comparative susceptibility of *Mycoplasma pneumoniae* to erythromycin, ciprofloxacin and lomefloxacin. Diagn Microbiol Infect Dis 1989;12:433.

10. Smith CB, Friedewald WT, Chanock RM. Shedding of *Mycoplasma pneumoniae* after tetracycline and erythromycin therapy. N Engl J Med 1967;276:1172.

11. Grayston JT, Kuo C-C, Wang S-P, et al. A new *Chlamydia psittaci* strain, TWAR, isolated in acute respiratory tract infections. N Engl J Med 1986;315:161.

12. Hahn DL, Dodge RW, Golubjatnikov R. Association of *Chlamydia pneumoniae* (strain TWAR) infection with wheezing, asthmatic bronchitis, and adult-onset asthma. JAMA 1991;266:225.

13. Grayston JT, Diwan VK, Cooney M, et al. Community- and hospital-acquired pneumonia associated with Chlamydia TWAR infection demonstrated serologically. Arch Intern Med 1989;149:169.

14. Hammerschlag MR, Chirgwin K, Roblin PM, et al. Persistent infection with *Chlamydia pneumoniae* following acute respiratory illness. Clin Infect Dis 1992;14:178.

15. Campbell LA, Perez-Melgosa M, Hamilton DJ, et al. Detection of *Chlamydia pneumoniae* by polymerase chain reaction. J Clin Microbiol 1992;30:434.

16. Gaydos CA, Quinn TC, Eiden JJ. Identification of *Chlamydia pneumoniae* by DNA amplification of the 16S rRNA gene. J Clin Microbiol 1992;30:796.

17. Kuo C-C, Grayston JT: In vitro drug susceptibility of Chlamydia sp. strain TWAR. Antimicrob Agents Chemother 1988;32:257.

18. Farizo KM, Cochi SL, Zell ER, et al. Epidemiological features of pertussis in the United States, 1980–1989. Clin Infect Dis 1992;14:708.

19. Christie CDC, Marx ML, Marchant CD, et al. The 1993 epidemic of pertussis in Cincinnati. N Engl J Med 1994;331:16.

20. Nennig ME, Shinefield HR, Edwards KM, et al. Prevalence and incidence of adult pertussis in an urban population. JAMA 1996;275:1672.

21. Henkinson D. Duration of effectiveness of pertussis vaccine: evidence from a 10-year community study. BMJ 1988;296:612.

22. Postels-Multani S, Schmitt HJ, Wirsing von Konig CH, et al. Symptoms and complications of pertussis in adults. Infection 1995;23:139.

23. Hoppe JE. Methods for isolation of *Bordetella pertussis* from patients with whooping cough. Euro J Clin Microbiol Infect Dis 1988;7:616.

24. Meade BD, Bollen A. Recommendations for use of the polymerase chain reaction in the diagnosis of *Bordetella pertussis* infections. J Med Microbiol 1994;41:51.

25. Bergquist SO, Bernander S, Dahnsjo H, et al. Erythromycin in the treatment of pertussis: a study of bacteriologic and clinical effects. Pediatr Infect Dis J 1987;6:458.

26. Shortridge KF. The next pandemic influenza virus? Lancet 1995;346:1210.

27. Sullivan KM, Monto AS, Longini IM Jr. Estimates of the U.S. health impact of influenza. Am J Public Health 1993;83:1712.

28. Lui KJ, Kendal AP. Impact of influenza epidemics on mortality in the United States from October 1972 to May 1985. Am J Public Health 1987;77:712.

29. Centers for Disease Control. Update: influenza activity—United States, 1996–97 season. MMWR 1997;46:76.

30. Gross PA. Preparing for the next influenza pandemic: a reemerging infection. Ann Intern Med 1996;124:682.

31. LaForce FM, Nichol KL, Cox NJ. Influenza: virology, epidemiology, disease, and prevention. Am J Prev Med 1994;10(Suppl):31.

32. ACIP. Prevention and control of influenza: recommendations of the Advisory Committee on Immunization Practices (ACIP). MMWR 1995;44(no. RR-3).

33. Thompson J, Fleet W, Lawrence E, et al. A comparison of acetaminophen and rimantadine in the treatment of influenza A in children. J Med Virol 1987;21:249.

34. Hayden FG, Belshe RB, Clover RD, et al. Emergence and apparent transmission of rimantadine-resistant influenza A virus in families. N Engl J Med 1989;321:1696.

35. Little JW, Hall WJ, Douglas RG Jr, et al. Airway hyperactivity and peripheral airway dysfunction in influenza A infection. Am Rev Repir Dis 1978;118:295.

36. Horner GJ, Gray FD Jr. Effect of uncomplicated presumptive influenza on the diffusing capacity of the lung. Am Rev Respir Dis 1973;108:866.

37. Foy HM, Cooney MK, Allen T, et al. Rates of pneumonia during influenza epidemics in Seattle, 1964 to 1975. JAMA 1979;241:253.

38. Louria DB, Blumenfeld HL, Ellis JT, et al. Studies on influenza in the pandemic of 1957–1958. II. Pulmonary complications of influenza. J Clin Invest 1959;38:213.

39. Martin LM, Kunin CM, Gottlieb LS, et al. Asian influenza A in Boston, 1957–1958. II. Severe staphylococcal pneumonia complicating influenza. Arch Intern Med 1959;103:532.

40. Schwarzmann SW, Adler JL, Sullivan RJ, et al. Bacterial pneumonia during the Hong Kong influenza epidemic of 1968–1969. Arch Intern Med 1971;127:1037.

41. Minow RA, Gorbach S, Johnson BL, et al. Myoglobinuria associated with influenza A infection. Ann Intern Med 1974; 80:359.

42. Greco TP, Askenase PW, Kashgarian M. Postviral myositis: myxovirus-like structures in affected muscle. Ann Intern Med 1977;86:193.

43. Hildebrandt HM, Maasab HF, Willis PW. Influenza virus pericarditis. Am J Dis Child 1962;104:179.

44. Adams CW. Post viral myopericarditis associated with influenza virus: report of eight cases. Am J Cardiol 1959;4:56.

45. Sperber SJ, Francis JB. Toxic shock during an influenza outbreak. JAMA 1987;257:1086.

46. Wells CEC, James WRL, Evans AD. Guillain-Barré syndrome and virus of influenza A (Asian strain). Arch Neurol Psychiatr 1959;81:699.

47. Wells CEC. Neurologic complications of so-called influenza: a winter study in southeast Wales. BMJ 1971;1:369.

48. Bayer WH. Influenza B encephalitis. West J Med 1987;147:466.

49. Corey L, Rubin RJ, Hattwick MA, et al. A nationwide outbreak of Reye's syndrome: its epidemiologic relationship to influenza B. Am J Med 1976;61:615.

50. Gwaltney JM, Jr, Phillips CD, Miller RD, et al. Computed tomographic study of the common cold. N Engl J Med 1994;330:25.

51. Franks P, Gleiner JA. The treatment of acute bronchitis with trimethoprim and sulfamethoxazole. J Fam Pract 1984;19:185.

52. Verheij TJM, Hermans J, Mulder JD. Effects of doxycycline in patients with acute cough and purulent sputum: a double-blind placebo-controlled study. Br J Gen Pract 1994;44:400.

53. Gonzales R, Sande M. What will it take to stop physicians from prescribing antibiotics in acute bronchitis. Lancet 1995;345:665–666.

54. Orr PH, Scherer K, MacDonald A, et al. Randomized placebo-controlled trials of antibiotic for acute bronchitis: a critical review of the literature. J Fam Pract 1993;36:507.

55. Henry D, Ruoff GE, Rhudy J. Effectiveness of short-course therapy with cefuroxime axetil in treatment of secondary bacterial infections of acute bronchitis. Antimicrob Agents Chemother 1995;39:2528

56. Comacho AE, Cobo R, Otte J, et al. Clinical comparison of cefuroxime axetil and amoxicillin/clavulanate in the treatment of patients with acute bacterial maxillary sinusitis. Am J Med 1992;93:271.

57. Nolen TM, Phillips HL, Hutchison J, et al. Comparison of cefuroxime axetil and cefaclor for patients with lower respiratory tract infections presenting to a rural family practice clinic. Curr Ther Res Clin Exp 1988;44:821.

58. Schleupner CJ, Anthony WC, Tan J, et al. Blinded comparison of cefuroxime to cefaclor for lower respiratory tract infections. Arch Intern Med 1988;148:343.

59. Snider GL. Emphysema: the first two centuries—and beyond. Am Rev Respir Dis 1992;146(Part I):1334.

60. Burrows B, Bloom JW, Traver GA, et al. The course and prognosis of different forms of chronic airways obstruction in a sample from the general population. N Engl J Med 1987; 317:1309.

61. Petty TL. Definitions in chronic obstructive pulmonary disease. Clin Chest Med 1990;11:363.

62. American Thoracic Society. Standards for the diagnosis and care of patients with chronic obstructive pulmonary disease (COPD) and asthma. Am Rev Resp Dis 1987;136:225.

63. Minette A. Is chronic bronchitis also an industrial disease? Eur J Respir Dis 1986;69(Suppl 146):87.

64. Speizer FE, Tager B. Epidemiology of chronic mucus hypersecretion and obstructive airways disease. Epidemiol Rev 1979;1:124.

65. Eadie MB, Stott EJ, Grist NR. Virological studies in chronic bronchitis. BMJ 1966;2:671.

66. Gump DW, Phillips CA, Forsyth BR, et al. Role of infection in chronic bronchitis. Am Rev Respir Dis 1976;113:465.

67. Lamy ME, Pouthier-Simon F, Debacker-Willame E. Respiratory viral infections in hospital patients with chronic bronchitis. Chest 1973;63:336.

68. McNamara MJ, Phillips IA, Williams OB. Viral and *Mycoplasma pneumoniae* infections in exacerbations of chronic lung disease. Am Rev Respir Dis 1969;100:19.

69. Stark JE, Heath RB, Curwen MP. Infection with parainfluenza viruses in chronic bronchitis. Thorax 1965;20:124.

70. Buscho RO, Saxtan D, Shultz PS, et al. Infections with viruses and *Mycoplasma pneumoniae* during exacerbations of chronic bronchitis. J Infect Dis 1978;1378:377.

71. Carilli AD, Gohd RS, Gordon W. A virologic study of chronic bronchitis. N Engl J Med 1964;270:123.

72. Chodosh S. Treatment of acute exacerbations of chronic bronchitis: state of the art. Am J Med 1991;91(Suppl 6A):87S.

73. Chodosh S. Examination of sputum cells. N Engl J Med 1970;282:854.

74. Fournier M, Lebargy F, Leroy Ladurie F, et al. Intraepithelial T-lymphocyte subsets in the airways of normal subjects and/or patients with chronic bronchitis. Am Rev Respir Dis 1989;140:737.

75. Saetta M, DiStefano A, Maestrelli P, et al. Activated T-lymphocytes and macrophages in bronchial mucosa of subjects with chronic bronchitis. Am Rev Respir Dis 1993;147:301.

76. Dunnill MS, Massarella GR, Anderson JA. A comparison of the quantitative anatomy of the bronchi in normal subjects, in status asthmaticus, in chronic bronchitis, and in emphysema. Thorax 1969;24:176.

77. Lees AW, McNaught W. Bacteriology of lower respiratory tract secretions, sputum, and upper respiratory tract secretions in "normals" and chronic bronchitis. Lancet 1959;2:1112.

78. Miller DL, Jones R. The bacterial flora of the upper respiratory tract and sputum of working men. J Pathol Bacteriol 1964;87:182.

79. Murphy TF, Apicella MA. Nontypable *Hemophilus influenzae:* a review of clinical aspects, surface antigens, and the human immune response to infection. Rev Infect Dis 1987;9:1.

80. Bjerkestrand G, Digranes A, Schreiner A. Bacteriological findings in transtracheal aspirates from patients with chronic bronchitis and bronchiectasis. Scand J Resp Dis 1975;56:201.

81. Bartlett J. Diagnostic accuracy of transtracheal aspiration bacteriologic studies. Am Rev Respir Dis 1977;115:777.

82. Rodnick JE, Gude JK. The use of antibiotics in acute bronchitis and acute exacerbations of chronic bronchitis. West J Med 1988;149:347.

83. Murphy TF, Sethi S. Bacterial infection in chronic obstructive pulmonary disease. Am Rev Respir Dis 1992;146:1067.

84. Saint S, Bent S, Vittinghoff E, et al. Antibiotics in chronic obstructive pulmonary disease exacerbations: a meta-analysis. JAMA 1995;273:957.

85. Anthonisen NR, Manfreda J, Warren CPW, et al. Antibiotic therapy in exacerbations of chronic obstructive pulmonary disease. Ann Intern Med 1987;106:196.

86. Elmes PC, Fletcher CM, Dutton AAC. Prophylactic use of oxytetracycline for exacerbations of chronic bronchitis. BMJ 1957;2:1272.

87. Elmes PC, King TKC, Langlands JHM, et al. Value of ampicillin in the hospital treatment of exacerbations of chronic bronchitis. BMJ 1965;2:904.

88. Nicotra MB, Rivera M, Awe RJ. Antibiotic therapy of acute exacerbations of chronic bronchitis. Ann Intern Med 1982;97:18.

89. Pines A, Raafat H, Plucinski K, et al. Antibiotic regimens in severe and acute purulent exacerbations of chronic bronchitis. BMJ 1968;2:735.

90. Berry DG, Fry J, Hindley CP, et al. Exacerbations of chronic bronchitis treatment with oxytetracycline. Lancet 1960;1:137.

91. Fear EC, Edwards G. Antibiotic regimes in chronic bronchitis. Br J Dis Chest 1962;56:153.

92. Petersen ES, Esmann V, Honcke P, et al. A controlled study of the effect of treatment on chronic bronchitis: an evaluation using pulmonary function tests. Acta Med Scand 1967;182:293.

93. Jorgensen AF, Coolidge J, Pedersen PA, et al. Amoxicillin in treatment of acute uncomplicated exacerbations of chronic bronchitis. Scand J Prev Health Care 1992;10:7.

94. Ziment I. Pharmacologic therapy of obstructive airway disease. Clin Chest Med 1990;11:461.

95. Nichol KL, Lind A, Margolis KL, et al. The cost effectiveness of vaccination against influenza in healthy, working adults. N Engl J Med 1995;333:889.

96. Shapiro ED, Berg AT, Austrian R, et al. The protective efficacy of polyvalent pneumococcal polysaccharide vaccine. N Engl J Med 1991;325:1453.

97. Centers for Disease Control. Pneumococcal polysaccharide vaccine. MMWR 1989;38:68.

98. Johnston RN, McNeill RS, Smith DH, et al. Five-year winter chemoprophylaxis for chronic bronchitis. BMJ 1969;4:265.

99. Medical Research Council Working Party on Trials of Chemotherapy in Early Chronic Bronchitis. Value of chemoprophylaxis and chemotherapy in early chronic bronchitis. BMJ 1966;1:317.

100. Pridie RB, Datta N, Massey DG, et al. A trial of continuous winter chemotherapy in chronic bronchitis. Lancet 1960;2:723.

101. Amer Rev Resp Dis 1990;141:642.

102. Mello CJ, Irwin RS, Curley FJ. Predictive values of the character, timing, and complications of chronic cough in diagnosing its cause. Arch Intern Med 1996;156:997.

CHAPTER 3

The Common Cold

John G. Bartlett

Snapshot Summary

Etiology
   Most common: Rhinovirus and coronavirus.
   Also: Parainfluenza virus, respiratory syncytial virus
      (RSV), adenovirus, and influenza.
   Treatable and rare: *Mycoplasma pneumoniae* and
      Chlamydia pneumoniae.
Differential diagnosis (major alternative diagnoses)
   Allergic rhinitis: Nasal obstruction, sneezing, nasal pru-
      ritus, eye irritation or pruritus, and lacrimation, often
      seasonal or with exposures. Nasal drainage shows
      eosinophils; nasal membranes are bluish and boggy.
   Vasomotor rhinitis: Nasal obstruction and drainage
      without pruritus or atopy.
Transmission of cold viruses: Primarily by hand contact.
Complications:
   Contiguous infections: Sinusitis, bronchitis, otitis.
   Pulmonary: Exacerbations of chronic bronchitis,
      asthma, pneumonia, obstructive sleep apnea.
   Functional capacity: Reduce pulmonary function for
      weeks.

Treatment

Recommended: Ipratropium bromide spray, nonsteroidal anti-inflammatory agents.

Possibly effective: Zinc gluconate lozenges, antihistamines (especially sedating first generation agents).

Not recommended: Oral decongestants, antibacterial agents, vitamin C, heated humidified air, or intranasal steroids.

Allergic rhinitis: Antihistamines and intranasal steroids are highly effective.

The common cold is a relatively mild illness, but it has an extraordinary impact on medical practice, absenteeism, and economic consequences due to work loss. Virtually everyone is an "expert" on the common cold because of first-hand experience—again, again, and again. Nevertheless, this is one of those common conditions in medicine where substantial misinformation exists about both epidemiology and treatment.

Impact

The common cold is a major cause of morbidity in terms of work loss and school absenteeism (Table 3.1). Common secondary complications include otitis, sinusitis, laryngitis, chronic bronchitis exacerbations, and asthma. The estimated economic burden in the United States exceeds $2 billion per year in cold remedies and physician visits (1–3), which equates to about $10 per person per year.

Etiology

A variety of conditions can cause symptoms of the common cold, but this term is usually reserved for those caused by an upper respiratory tract viral infection (Table 3.2).

Table 3.1
Consequences of the Common Cold
in the United States (1–3)

Acute disabling illnesses:	20%
Restricted activity:	170,000,000 days/year (0.8 days/person)
Physician contact:	22,000,000 (10% of population)
Loss of work:	30,000,000 days/year
School absenteeism:	30,000,000 days/year
Physician-related expenses:	$1.5 billion/year ($6/person)
Cold remedies (nonprescription drugs):	$1 billion/year ($4/person)

Table 3.2
Causes of Common Cold Symptoms

Viruses that cause the common cold

MOST FREQUENT
  Rhinovirus   Influenza
  Coronavirus   Parainfluenza

LESS COMMON
  Respiratory syncytial   Enterovirus
    virus   Reovirus
  Adenovirus   Picornaviruses

Other conditions that cause common cold symptoms

INFECTIONS
  Mycoplasma pneumoniae
  Chlamydia pneumoniae

NONINFECTIOUS DISEASES
  Vasomotor rhinitis   Nasal septal defects
  Allergic rhinitis   Prior nasal surgery
  Atrophic rhinitis   Foreign bodies
  Nasal polyposis   Nasal neoplasms
  Gustatory rhinitis

Rhinovirus is the most common viral agent. More than 100 serologic types of rhinovirus exist, which partially explains the probability of multiple infections by this class of organisms. In addition, symptom variations exist that, presumably, are based on partial immunity. Although rhinoviruses are most common, they actually account for only 25%–40% of cases of the common cold (4–8).

Coronaviruses are also common causes of colds, but are less well studied because they are difficult to cultivate. Other relatively common viral pathogens of the upper airways are adenovirus, parainfluenza virus, respiratory syncytial virus (RSV), and influenza virus. Influenza causes common cold symptoms, but systemic response is usually profound so that "flu" is usually distinguishable from a "cold." RSV is an important cause of potentially serious disease in children. In adults, RSV usually causes a common cold, but the disease may be serious in the elderly and in immunocompromised patients. Parainfluenza virus is another common cause of lower respiratory tract infections in children that causes the common cold, often with hoarseness, in adults. Pharyngeal infections caused by *Mycobacterium pneumoniae, Chlamydia pneumoniae,* or Streptococci (group A, C, or G) may cause symptoms of the common cold, but they are infrequent. Common noninfectious diseases associated with cold symptoms are described below.

Rhinovirus Infection

The best studied agent of the common cold is rhinovirus, which was first detected in 1956 (9). The nose or eye, not the mouth, is the usual portal of entry; transmission is usually by hand contact (10,11). The nasopharynx appears to be the initial site of infection. The M cells in lymphoepithelial regions of the adenoids contain the ICAM-1 receptors for rhinovirus (9,12–14). The virus presumably reaches the posterior nasopharynx by mucociliary activity in the nose which carries the nasal mucus to the adenoidal crypts (12). The infection then spreads anteriorly to the nasal passages. Once the infection is established, the virus replicates to reach a peak concentration at 48 hours (12,15). Viral shedding persists up to 3 weeks. It is not known whether rhinovirus infects cells of the lower airways, but the optimal temperature for its replication is 33°C, which is readily achieved in nasal passages. Biopsies of nasal epithelium show infected cells, but no cytopathology (12), suggesting other mechanisms are responsible for clinical symptoms. Postulated mechanisms are inflammatory mediators and neurologic reflexes. The candidate inflammatory mediators include kinins (bradykinin and iyslbradykinin), interleukin 1 and 8, selected prostaglandins, and histamine (9,16,17). Support for these inflammatory mediators' role is based on their detection in increased concentrations in nasal secretions that accompany the common cold due to rhinovirus (9). The role of histamine is unclear: intranasal instillation of histamine causes symptoms of the common cold, but the results of therapeutic trials with antihistamines are variable (16,17). A parasympathetic block reduces symptoms of the common cold, suggesting a role for neurologic reflexes (18).

Symptoms of the common cold include nasal drainage, nasal obstruction, sneezing, and coughing. The physiologic basis for these symptoms appears to be vasodilation and glandular secretion. Recent studies indicate that rhinovirus and colds due to other viruses are usually associated with infundibular occlusion of sinuses with sinusitis (19). This observation suggests the term "rhinosinusitis" is more appropriate than "rhinitis" (9). However, it is important to emphasize that implications for therapy are unchanged by this observation because patients in this study had spontaneous resolution of computed tomography (CT) scan evidence for sinusitis.

Noninfectious Diseases Associated with Cold Symptoms

ALLERGIC RHINITIS

Allergic rhinitis is the most common allergic condition; it affects more than 20 million persons in the United States (20). Typical symptoms are nasal obstruction, sneezing, and nasal pruritus. Associated symptoms include eye irritation or pruritus and lacrimation. Common complications include eustachian tube blockage with serous otitis, asthma, sinusitis, and postnasal drainage with cough or bronchitis. These symptoms may be seasonal or perennial, and the precipitating cause is exposure to common allergens such as animal dander or pollens. Physical examination of the nasal mucosa shows it to be pale, boggy, and bluish. The nasal discharge, which is clear or slightly discolored, shows eosinophils on microscopic examination. Recommended treatment includes antihistamines, cromoglycate, systemic decongestants, and corticosteroid nasal sprays. Intranasal corticosteroids are the most effective of these (20). Severe cases are often managed with allergy skin testing and immunotherapy. Some cases in which no history of an atopy exists and skin tests are negative are managed as described above, but without immunotherapy.

VASOMOTOR RHINITIS

Typical symptoms of vasomotor rhinitis are nasal obstruction, nasal drainage, and postnasal drainage without pruritus or atopy. The precipitating cause appears to be nonspecific irritants such as fumes, temperature changes, humidity, or air conditioning. Treatment is with antihistamines, systemic decongestants, and corticosteroid nasal sprays.

ATROPHIC RHINITIS

Atrophic rhinitis is characterized by atrophy of the nasal mucosa and adjacent structures. Typical symptoms are nasal crusting, foul-smelling drainage, and loss of smell and taste. Purulent drainage usually indicates a superimposed bacterial infection. Occasionally, patients have vitamin A or iron deficiencies, and some have infections involving *Klebsiella ozaenae*. Prior nasal or sinus surgery may also cause this complication. Treatment consists of daily irrigations with saline and nasal moisturizers. Antibiotics are advocated for exacerbations associated with purulent drainage.

NASAL POLYPOSIS

Nasal polyposis is a grapelike mass in the nose that usually arises from paranasal sinuses. Some cases represent complications of chronic sinus infections; others are associated with asthma or cystic fibrosis. A common complication is sinusitis. Treatment consists of intranasal corticosteroids, short-term systemic corticosteroids, and antibiotic treatment of sinusitis. Endoscopic sinus surgery is sometimes required.

GUSTATORY RHINITIS

The term "gustatory rhinitis" refers to rhinorrhea associated with eating hot or spicy foods. It results from parasympathetic response and may be reversed with intranasal anticholinergics.

Epidemiology

The number of colds decreases with age. Preschool children average four to eight colds per year, school age children average two to six per year, and adults average two to five per year (21–24). The frequency is increased among persons living in crowded conditions and among mothers with young children (4). In temperate climates, the risk is greatest in the colder months; this especially applies to infections with coronavirus, RSV, and influenza (8,25). The association of upper respiratory tract infections (URIs) with the winter season account for the term "common cold," but cold weather, chilling, and dampness have no impact on susceptibility per se (26,27); the association with cold weather presumably reflects promotion of contact owing to indoor clustering within families, day care settings, schools, and military groups. Persons who smoke are more likely to acquire a cold and to have more severe symptoms (28,29). Psychological stress also appears to play a role: Studies in volunteers challenged with rhinovirus types 2, 9, or 14; coronavirus type 229E; or RSV indicate psychological stress increased susceptibility in a dose-response relationship (30). The multitude of colds during the lifetime of any individual reflects the facts that there are more than 200 types of viruses that cause colds (see Table 3.2), and that many respiratory viruses result in only transient immunity so that reinfection with some viruses (RSV, parainfluenza, and coronaviruses) is common (5,30,31).

Transmission

Transmission of viruses that cause the common cold is primarily by direct contact with respiratory secretions. The usual mechanism is hand contact with an infected individual or contaminated object, followed by self-inoculation by either finger-to-nose or finger-to-eye spread (32–34). It appears that transmission by air is not efficient for most viruses and even "wet kissing" is less efficient compared with hand contact (35). Aerosol spread appears important in the transmission of influenza virus and some picornaviruses (36).

Clinical Features

Symptoms are well known to everyone. The incubation period is 2–4 days at which time the virus is primarily in the ciliated epithelium of the nose. The initial clinical symptoms are related to nasal passages with rhinorrhea, sneezing, nasal obstruction, and postnasal drip. Other common symptoms include sore throat, throat clearing, hoarseness, and cough. Systemic symptoms are variable, but many patients experience malaise and myalgia and sometimes low-grade fever. Pathologic studies show minimal damage to the nasal mucosa (37,38); it appears that the clinical expression is chemically or neurologically mediated as summarized above (39–42). Illness severity reflects viral shedding, which is maximal at an average of 48 hours, and then resolves. Immune defenses produce interferon (which may account for systemic complaints) and then secretory IgA. The median duration of symptoms is 7–13 days (43). Viral shedding may last 14–21 days; focal areas of distorted nasal mucosal cilia may persist for 2–10 weeks (44).

Treatment

Few conditions in medicine have so many therapeutic options that do not work. Those with probable benefit for the common cold are largely limited to intranasal ipratropism bromide and analgesics (Tables 3.3 and 3.4).

Intranasal anticholinergics (ipratropium bromide nasal spray) have demonstrated benefit in placebo-controlled trials for reduction in nasal drainage as measured by weighing used nasal tissue and reduction in sneezing (18,20,45). Symptom relief is better with treatment initiated within 1 day. The major side effect is blood-tinged mucus in 15%–20% of patients.

Table 3.3
Treatment of the Common Cold

Agent	Response
Intranasal ipratropium bromide	Reduced rhinorrhea and decreased sneezing, especially if initiated within 1 day
Cromoglycate—intranasal	No benefit except with allergic rhinitis; main benefit is to protect against airway response with allergen exposure (20)
Corticosteroids—intranasal	No benefit except with allergic rhinitis (20)
Corticosteroids—systemic	Should be reserved for severe cases of allergic rhinitis, nasal polyposis with obstruction, and rhinitis medicamentosa (20)
Aspirin and acetaminophen	Variable effect on nasal symptoms, suppressed antibody response, and prolonged viral shedding (46,47)
Ibuprofen	Symptomatic relief (46–52)
Nasal decongestants	May improve sleep Excessive use—"rebound nasal congestion" or "rhinitis medicamentosa"
Oral decongestants	Questionable benefit (49–52)
Antihistamines	Major benefit with allergic rhinitis Results with rhinovirus infection show reduced sneezing and rhinorrhea; there may be a difference between 1st generation antihistamines vs. nonsedating antihistamines favoring the former (20, 51–55)
Antibiotics	Possible benefit in 20% who are colonized with *Staphylococcus pneumoniae, Hemophilus influenzae,* or *Morexella catarrhalis,* and in rare cases involving *Mycoplasma pneumoniae* or *Chlamydia pneumoniae* (56–62)

(continued)

Table 3.3 *(continued)*

Agent	Response
Vitamin C	Variable results, but some studies show duration and severity of cold may be decreased (64–68)
Zinc gluconate lozenges	Variable results (69–74); controlled trials show inconsistent reduction in duration of symptoms, but results are inconsistent, rationale is unclear and side effects are common
Interferon alpha 2b	Clinical response with intranasal application but not realistic for routine use (77)
Humidified hot air	Rationale is to inhibit rhinovirus which grows optimally at 33°C; therapeutic trials show no benefit (75–76)

Aspirin, acetaminophen, and ibuprofen provide symptomatic relief, although aspirin may be associated with increased shedding of rhinovirus (20,46–48).

Nasal decongestants may help the patient sleep. However, because excessive use can result in "rebound" congestion nasal decongestants should be limited to 3–5 days. Oral decongestants are probably not effective and their use is complicated by side effects (20,49–51).

Antihistamines (first generation) reduce sneezing and nasal drainage (16,52–55). Nonsedating antihistamines lack anticholinergic activity and show variable results.

Antibacterial agents are also commonly prescribed, but they have no established benefit either for treatment or for prophylaxis to prevent common complications such as sinusitis (56–58). A possible exception is based on a recent

Table 3.4
Medications Commonly Used for URIs and Allergic Rhinitis[a]

Agent	Regimen	Cost[b]	Comment
Anticholinergics Ipratropium 0.3% (Atrovent)	2 sprays bid or tid	$33/30 mL	
Nasal decongestants Pseudoephedrine[b]	30 mg po bid	$0.03/30 mg	Commonly included in combinations with antihistamines and mucolytics
Zinc gluconate lozenges (Cold-Eze)	13.3–23 mg zn lozenge q2h while awake		Available in health food stores and pharmacies
Intranasal corticosteroids Flunisolide (Nasalide)	2 sprays bid	$27/25 mL	About 10% experience nasal irritation
Beclomethasone (Beconase AQ)	2 sprays bid	$35/25 g	
Triamcinolone (Nasacort)	2 sprays daily	$37/10 g	
Budesonide (Rhinocort)	2 sprays bid	$31/7 g	
Fluticasone (Flonase)	2 sprays daily	$31/9 g	

[a] Adapted from: Guarderas JC. Rhinitis and sinusitis: office management. Mayo Clin Proc 1996;71:882.
[b] Medi-span. Hospital Formulary Pricing Guide, Indianapolis, IN, January, 1997.

(continued)

Table 3.4 *(continued)*			
Agent	Regimen	Cost[b]	Comment
Cromoglycate (Nasalcrom)[b]	1 spray qid	$0.07/2 mL	
Antihistamine			
Diphenhydramine (Benadryl)[b]	25 mg q8h		Avoid use of astemizole with macrolides and imidazoles (ketoconazole, itraconazole, fluconazole, erythromycin, clarithromycin)
Astemizole (Hismanal)	10 mg daily	$1.92/10 mg	
Loratadine (Claritin)	10 mg daily	$2.02/10 mg	
Hydroxyzine (Atarax)[b]	25 mg qid	$0.03/25 mg	Nonsedating agents are astemizole, fexofenadine, and loratadine
Acrivastine (Semprex-D)	8 mg qid	$0.56/8 mg	
Fexofenadine (Allegra)	60 mg bid	$0.86/60 mg	Limit use to 3–5 days
Vasoconstrictors			
Oxyonetazone nasal solution (0.05%) (Afrin, Allerest, Dristan, Neo-Synephrine, NZT)	2–3 qtts each nostril bid		

placebo-controlled trial of 300 patients who had typical, uncomplicated URIs with nasal congestion, rhinorrhea, or pharyngitis. Participants had bacterial cultures of naso-pharyngeal washings and were randomized to receive amoxicillin-clavulanate (375 mg three times daily for 5 days) or placebo. In the subgroup of 61 (20%) who had cultures yielding *Streptococcus pneumoniae, Hemophilus influenzae,* or *Moraxella catarrhalis,* significant improvement was seen in symptom scores in those given the antibiotic. Similar results were noted in an earlier study of 507 patients (60); here the benefit was in a subset with nasopharyngeal secretions showing leukocytes and bacterial pathogens. Most authorities conclude that the risk of antibiotic resistance outweighs the modest benefit noted in these studies, although some have suggested limiting treatment to those with leukocytes in respiratory secretions (61).

Antiviral agents are generally not available for the agents of the common cold except amantadine and rimantadine for influenza A (if given within 48 hours of onset of symptoms). Ribavarin in active versus influenza A and B, RSV, and parainfluenza virus, but its use is limited to pediatric patients with RSV lower respiratory tract infections.

Vitamin C was once the subject of substantial controversy that, in part, reflected the stature of its advocate, Linus Pauling (64). Controlled trials have shown variable results, but most authorities conclude it plays no clear role in the treatment or prevention of common colds (65–68).

Zinc gluconate lozenges may reduce common cold symptoms' duration (69–71), although the results are inconsistent (72–74). A possible mechanism is that zinc ions inhibit common cold virus replication. However, the physiology of this benefit is anatomically enigmatic because the viruses that cause URIs are in the nose and the zinc lozenges are used in the oral cavity. No impact on viral shedding has been noted (74). Side effects include nausea and an unpleasant taste.

Heated humidified air is attractive as a method to inhibit the rhinovirus, which replicates optimally at 33°C. The original study of efficacy showed rapid subjective response (75). Subsequent studies have shown no beneficial effect (76).

Conclusions from this review are that a limited number of drugs have documented benefit. Intranasal ipratropium bromide has established merit for reducing rhinorrhea, especially if initiated early in the course of symptoms. Aspirin, acetaminophen, and ibuprofen may be given for symptomatic relief. Nasal decongestants can be provided to improve sleep. Zinc gluconate lozenges may reduce the duration of symptoms, but the benefit in clinical trials is inconsistent. Other drugs have no established merit despite extensive use. A critical component in the assessment is to distinguish those patients with allergic rhinitis who will benefit from intranasal corticosteroids and antihistamines.

Complications

Two types of complications (Table 3.5) exist. One consists of infections, often due to bacteria, at contiguous sites such as sinusitis, otitis media, bronchitis, and pneumonia (20,77,78). The second concerns lung disease. Common colds are associated with exacerbations of chronic obstructive pulmonary disease, asthma, and obstructive sleep apnea (79–82). Most patients with common colds that persist longer than 48 hours have sinusitis as detected by CT scan (19). These changes clear without antibiotic treatment according to follow-up scans at 2–3 weeks. Some studies show that about 2% of colds are complicated by sinusitis sufficiently severe to merit antibacterial treatment (see Chapter 5, Sinusitis). Many patients with the common cold have abnormal pulmonary function tests, including decreased diffusing capacity, reduced inspiratory flow rates, and increased closing volume (83).

Table 3.5
Complications of the Common Cold

Infections of contiguous sites (75)

Sinusitis	Pneumonia
Otitis media	Bronchitis

Pulmonary complications

Asthma (76,77)
Exacerbation of chronic pulmonary disease (78)
Abnormal pulmonary function:
   Decreased diffusing capacity, decreased inspiratory flow
    rate, increased closing volume (79)
Obstructive sleep apnea (80)

Prevention

The most important preventive mechanism is avoidance of contact, especially hand contact, with patients with typical symptoms. Virucidal paper handkerchiefs and good personal hygiene have been shown to reduce transmission of experimental colds caused by rhinovirus (84). Vitamin C was often advocated as a method to prevent the common cold, but appropriately controlled trials have not supported this tactic (56,57). Interferon alpha-2b was effective as short-term prophylaxis, but concern exists about the side effects of nasal stuffiness, and this approach has been discontinued (85).

References

1. National Center for Health Statistics. Current estimates from the National Health Interview Survey, United States, 1988. DHHS Publication No. (PHS)88-1594.

2. Couch RB. The common cold: control? J Infect Dis 1984;150:167.

3. Lowenstein SR, Parrino TA. Management of the common cold. Adv Intern Med 1987;32:207.

4. Monto AS, Ullman BM. Acute respiratory illness in an American community. JAMA 1974;227:164.

5. Denny FW. Acute respiratory infections in children: etiology and epidemiology. Pediatr Rev 1987;9:135.

6. Higgins PG. Viruses associated with acute respiratory infections 1961–71. J Hyg (Camb) 1974;72:425.

7. Monto A. The common cold: cold water on hot news. JAMA 1994;271:1122.

8. Hall CB, McBride JT. Upper respiratory tract infections: the common cold, pharyngitis, croup, bacterial tracheitis and epiglottitis. In: Pennington J, ed. Respiratory infection: diagnosis and management, 3rd ed. New York: Raven Press, 1994; 101–123.

9. Gwaltney JM. Rhinovirus infection of the normal human airway. Am J Respir Crit Care Med 1995;152:536.

10. Bynoe ML, Hobson D, Horner J, et al. Inoculation of human volunteers with a strain of virus from a common cold. Lancet 1961;1:1194.

11. Douglas RG Jr. Pathogenesis of rhinovirus common colds in human volunteers. Ann Otol Rhinol Laryngol 1970;79:563.

12. Winther B, Gwaltney JM Jr, Mygind N, et al. Sites of recovery after point inoculation of the upper airway. JAMA 1986; 256:1763.

13. Winther B, Innes DJ. The human adenoid: a morphologic study. Arch Otolaryngol Head Neck Surg 1994;120:144.

14. Winther B, Innes DJ, Hendley JO, et al. Distribution of the human rhinovirus receptor, ICAM-1, on epithelium of the upper airways [abstract]. J Japan Rhinol Soc 1991;A100.

15. Douglas RG Jr, Cate TR, Gerone PJ, et al. Quantitative rhinovirus shedding patterns in volunteers. Am Rev Respir Dis 1966;94:159.

16. Doyle WJ, Boehm S, Skoner DP. Physiologic responses to intranasal dose-response challenges with histamine, methacholine, bradykinin, and prostaglandin in adult volunteers with and without nasal allergy. J Allergy Clin Immunol 1990;86:924.

17. Proud D, Gwaltney JM Jr, Hendley JO, et al. Increased levels of interleukin-1 are detected in nasal secretions of volunteers during experimental rhinovirus colds. J Infect Dis 1994;169:1007.

18. Gaffey MJ, Hayden FG, Boyd JC, et al. Ipratropium bromide treatment of experimental rhinovirus infection. Antimicrob Agents Chemother 1988;32:1644.

19. Gwaltney JM Jr, Phillips CD, Miller RD, et al. Computed tomographic study of the common cold. N Engl J Med 1994;330:25.

20. Guarderas JC. Rhinitis and sinusitis: office management. Mayo Clin Proc 1996;71:882.

21. Badger GF, Dingle JH, Feller AE. A study of illness in a group of Cleveland families. II. Incidence of common respiratory diseases. Am J Hyg 1953;41.

22. Brimblecombe FSW, Cruickshank R, Masters PL, et al. Family studies of respiratory infections. BM J 1958;1:119.

23. Fox JP, Hall CE, Cooney MK, et al. The Seattle virus watch. II. Objectives. Study population and its observation data processing and summary of illnesses. Am J Epidemiol 1972;96:270.

24. Gwaltney JM Jr, Hendley JO, Simon G, et al. Rhinovirus infections in an industrial population. I. The occurrence of illness. N Engl J Med 1966;275:1261.

25. Douglas RG Jr, Lindgren KM, Couch RB. Exposure to cold environment and rhinovirus common cold. N Engl J Med 1968;279:742.

26. Douglas RG Jr, Lindgren KM, Couch RB. Exposure to cold environment and rhinovirus common cold: failure to demonstrate effect. N Engl J Med 1968;279:743.

27. Couch RB. Rhinoviruses. In: Fields BN, ed. Virology. New York: Raven Press, 1985;795–816.

28. Aronson MD, Weiss ST, Ben RL, et al. Association between cigarette smoking and acute respiratory tract illness in young adults. JAMA 1982;248:181.

29. Blake GH, Abell TD, Stanley WG. Cigarette smoking and upper respiratory infection among recruits in basic combat training. Ann Intern Med 1988;109:198.

30. Cohen S, Tyrrell DAJ, Smith AP. Psychological stress and susceptibility to the common cold. N Engl J Med 1991;325:606.

31. Lowenstein SR, Parrino TA. Management of the common cold. Adv Intern Med 1987;32:207.

32. Gwaltney JM. Rhinovirus colds: epidemiology, clinical characteristics and transmission. Eur J Respir Dis 1983;64(Suppl 128):336.

33. Gwaltney JM Jr, Hendley JO. Rhinovirus transmission, one if by air, two if by hand. Am J Epidemiol 1978;107:357.

34. Hendley JO, Wentzel RP, Gwaltney JM Jr. Transmission of rhinovirus colds by self-inoculation. N Engl J Med 1973; 288:1361.

35. Peterson JA, D'Alessio DJ, Dick EC. Studies on the failure of direct oral contact to transmit rhinovirus infection between human volunteers. In: Abstracts of the Annual Meeting of the American Society for Microbiology. Miami: American Society for Microbiology, 1973;213.

36. Couch RB, Douglas RG Jr, Lindgren KM, et al. Airborne transmission of respiratory infection with coxsackie virus A type 21. Am J Epidemiol 1970;91:78.

37. Winther B, Gwaltney JM Jr, Hendley JO. Respiratory virus infection of monolayer cultures of human nasal epithelial cells. Am Rev Respir Dis 1990;141:839.

38. Winther B, Gwaltney JM Jr, Mygind N, et al. Site of rhinovirus recovery after point inoculation of the upper airway. JAMA 1986;256:1763.

39. Naclerio RM, Proud D, Lichtenstein LM, et al. Kinins are generated during experimental rhinovirus colds. J Infect Dis 1988;157:133.

40. Proud D, Naclerio RM, Gwaltney JM Jr, et al. Kinins are generated in nasal secretions during natural rhinovirus colds. J Infect Dis 1990;161:120.

41. Proud D, Reynolds CJ, Lacapra S, et al. Nasal provocation with bradykinin induces symptoms of rhinitis and a sore throat. Am Rev Respir Dis 1988;137:613.

42. Douglas RG Jr. Pathogenesis of rhinovirus common colds in human volunteers. Acta Otolaryngol (Stockh) 1970;79:563.

43. Monto AS, Bryan ER, Ohmit S. Rhinovirus infections in Tecumseh, Michigan: illness frequency and number of serotypes. J Infect Dis 1987;156:43.

44. Carson JL, Collier AM, Hu SS. Acquired ciliary defects in nasal epithelium of children with acute viral upper respiratory infections. N Engl J Med 1985;312:463.

45. Hayden FG, Diamond L, Wood PB, et al. Effectiveness and safety of intranasal ipratropium bromide in common colds. Ann Intern Med 1996;125:89.

46. Stanley ED, Jackson GG, Panusarn C, et al. Increased virus shedding with aspirin treatment of rhinovirus infection. JAMA 1975;231:1248.

47. Graham NMH, Burrell CJ, Douglas RM, et al. Adverse effects of aspirin, acetaminophen, and ibuprofen on immune function,

viral shedding, and clinical status in rhinovirus-infected volunteers. J Infect Dis 1990;162;1277.

48. Sperber SJ, Hendley JO, Hayden FG, et al. Effects of naproxen on experimental rhinovirus colds: a randomized, double-blind, controlled trial. Ann Intern Med 1992;117:37.

49. Hutton N, Wilson MH, Mellits ED, et al. Effectiveness of an antihistamine-decongestant combination for young children with the common cold: a randomized, controlled clinical trial. J Pediatr 1991;118:125.

50. Lampert RP, Robinson DS, Soyka LF. A critical look at oral decongestants. Pediatrics 1975;55:550.

51. Szilagyi PG. What can we do about the common cold? Contemporary Pediatrics 1990;7:23.

52. Smith MBH, Feldman W. Over-the-counter cold medications: a critical review of clinical trials between 1950 and 1991. JAMA 1993;269:2258.

53. Henauer SA, Gluck U. Efficacy of terfenadine in the treatment of common cold: a double-blind comparison with placebo. Eur J Clin Pharmacol 1988;34:35.

54. Berkowitz RB, Tinkelman DG. Evaluation of oral terfenadine for treatment of the common cold. Ann Allergy Asthma Immunol 1991;67:593.

55. West S, Brandon B, Stolley P, et al. A review of antihistamines and the common cold. Pediatrics 1975;56:100.

56. Gordon M, Lovell S, Dugdale AE. The value of antibiotics in minor respiratory illness in children. A controlled trial. Med J Aust 1974;1:304.

57. Soyka LF, Robinson DS, Lachant N, et al. The misuse of antibiotics for treatment of upper respiratory tract infections in children. Pediatrics 1975;55:552.

58. Schmidt JP, Metcalf TG, Miltenberger FW. An epidemic of Asian influenza in children at Ladd Air Force Base, Alaska, 1960. J Pediatr 1962;61:214.

59. Kaiser L, Lew D, Hirschel B, et al. Effects of antibiotic treatment in the subset of common cold patients who have bacteria in nasopharyngeal secretions. Lancet 1996;347:1507.

60. J Gen Intern Med 1993;8:667.

61. Trenholme GM. Effects of antibiotic treatment in the subset of common cold patients who have bacteria in nasopharyngeal secretions. Infect Dis Clin Pract 1996;5:421.

62. Wise R. Antibiotics for the uncommon cold. Lancet 1996;347:1499.

63. Centers for Disease Control and Prevention. Influenza: recommendations of the Advisory Council on Immunization Practices. MMWR 1995;44(RR-3):11.

64. Pauling LC. Vitamin C and the common cold. San Francisco: W.H. Freeman, 1970;26–38.

65. Coulehan JJ, Eberhard S, Kapner, et al. Vitamin C and acute illness in Navajo school children. N Engl J Med 1976;18:973.

66. Hemila H. Vitamin C and the common cold. Br J Nutr 1992;67:3.

67. Karlowski TR, Chalmers TC, Frenkel LD, et al. Ascorbic acid for the common cold. A prophylactic and therapeutic trial. JAMA 1975;231:1038.

68. Miller JZ, Nance WE, Norton JA, et al. Therapeutic effect of vitamin C: a co-twin control study. JAMA 1977;237:248.

69. Eby GA, Davis DR, Halcomb WW. Reduction in duration of common colds by zinc gluconate lozenges in a double-blind study. Antimicrob Agents Chemother 1984;25:20.

70. Mossad SB. Zinc gluconate lozenges for treating the common cold. A randomized, double-blind, placebo-controlled study. Ann Intern Med 1996;125:81.

71. Farr BM, Conner EM, Betts RF, et al. Two randomized controlled trials of zinc gluconate lozenge therapy of experimentally induced rhinovirus colds. Antimicrob Agents Chemother 1987;31:1183.

72. Weismann K, Jakobsen JP, Weismann JE, et al. Zinc gluconate lozenges for common cold. A double-blind clinical trial. Dan Med Bull 1990;37:279.

73. Smith DS, Helzner EC, Nuttall CE Jr, et al. Failure of zinc gluconate in treatment of acute upper respiratory tract infections. Antimicrob Agents Chemother 1989;33:646.

74. Zinc for the common cold. Med Lett Drugs Ther 1997;39:9.

75. Tyrrell DAJ. Hot news on the common cold. Ann Rev Microbiol 1988;42:35.

76. Forstall GJ, Macknin ML, Yen-Lieberman BR, et al. Effect of inhaling heated vapor on symptoms of the common cold. JAMA 1994;271:1109.

77. Gwaltney JM Jr. Combined antiviral and antimediator treatment of rhinovirus colds. J Infect Dis 1992;166:776.

78. Henderson FW, Collier AM, Sanyal MA, et al. Longitudinal study of respiratory viruses and bacteria in the etiology of acute otitis media with effusion. N Engl J Med 1982;306:1377.

79. Busse WW. Respiratory infections: their role in airway responsiveness and the pathogenesis of asthma. J Allergy Clin Immunol 1990;85:671.

80. Lemanske RFJ, Dick EC, Swenson CA, et al. Rhinovirus upper respiratory infection increases airway hyperactivity and late asthmatic reactions. J Clin Invest 1989;83:1.

81. Smith CB, Golden CA, Kanner RE, et al. Association of viral and mycoplasma pneumonial infections with acute respiratory illness in patients with chronic obstructive pulmonary diseases. Am Rev Respir Dis 1980;121:225.

82. Zwillich CW, Pickett C, Hanson FN, et al. Disturbed sleep and prolonged apnea during nasal obstruction in normal men. Am Rev Respir Dis 1981;124:158.

83. Hall WJ, Hall CB. Alterations in pulmonary function following respiratory viral infection. Chest 1979;76:458.

84. Dick EC, Hossain SU, Mink KA, et al. Interruption of transmission of rhinovirus colds among human volunteers using virucidal paper handkerchiefs. J Infect Dis 1986;153:352.

85. Monto AS, Schwartz SA, Albrecht JK. Ineffectiveness of post exposure prophylaxis of rhinovirus infection with low-dose intranasal alpha 2b interferon in families. Antimicrob Agents Chemother 1983;33:387.

86. Hayden FG, Albrecht JK, Kaiser DL, et al. Prevention of natural colds by contact prophylaxis with intranasal alpha interferon. N Engl J Med 1986;314:71.

Streptococcal Pharyngitis

John G. Bartlett

Snapshot Summary

Clinical features: Fever, sore throat, dysphagia, malaise, and headache.

Diagnosis

Throat culture: 90% sensitive, 96%–99% specific.

Rapid antigen detection: 30%–95% sensitive, 95%–100% specific.

Antibody response (antistreptolysin-O [ASLO]): 80% have fourfold increase.

Management recommendations

Supporting clinical features: Tonsillar exudate, tender cervical nodes, no cough, fever.

No. of possibilities	Probability of strep throat	Recommendation
0	2.5%	No culture, no treatment
1	6.5%	Culture, treat positives
2	15%	Culture, treat positives
3	32%	No culture, treat
4	56%	No culture, treat

Complications

 Suppurative complications: Peritonsillar abscess and
  suppurative adenitis.

 Epidemic spread.

 Nonsuppurative complications: Rheumatic fever, scarlet
  fever, glomerulonephritis, toxic shock syndrome.

Treatment

 Preferred: Penicillin for 10 days.

 Alternatives: Cephalosporins, macrolides (erythromycin),
  clindamycin.

 In the 1940s, throat culture evolved as a standard test
  to confirm the diagnosis of Streptococcal pharyngitis;
  penicillin became a well-established treatment, a
  10-day course of treatment proved necessary to eradicate group A beta-hemolytic Streptococci from the
  pharynx and the utility of this treatment to prevent
  rheumatic fever became well established (1–4). These
  principles still apply, although much has happened in
  the intervening four decades, suggesting that current
  management is as much art as science.

Epidemiology

Group A Streptococci causing pharyngitis are spread by
large airborne droplets. Fomites are not sources of pharyngitis. Factors that promote person-to-person transmission
include the number of organisms in the throat or nose,
virulence of the strain, and the closeness of contact. Host
susceptibility is unrelated to race, gender, socioeconomic
status, climate, or geography. In temperate climates, Streptococcal carriage and pharyngitis peak in the late winter
and early spring (5,6). Type-specific anti-M antibodies con-
fer protection for the homologous M type, but not to other
types. Transmission is much more efficient from symptomatic patients compared with colonized patients.

Clinical Presentation

Typical symptoms include the sudden onset of fever, chills without rigors, severe sore throat, dysphagia, malaise, and headache. Examination shows pharyngeal erythema or exudative pharyngitis and anterior cervical lymphadenopathy. Other findings often include petechiae on the soft palate and leukocytosis.

None of these clinical features are considered diagnostic of Streptococcal pharyngitis, but all are supportive or suggestive of it. Analysis of large numbers of patients for correlation between clinical observation and throat culture result show certain factors that are significantly associated with Streptococcal pharyngitis compared with viral pharyngitis. These include fever, absence of a cough, exposure to group A Streptococci, temperature higher than 38°C, pharyngeal inflammation, pharyngeal exudate, enlarged tonsils, palate petechiae, and anterior cervical lymphadenopathy (7). Rhinitis, laryngitis, and bronchitis are not features of Streptococcal pharyngitis, but they are common with viral pharyngitis. In general, clinicians overdiagnose Streptococcal pharyngitis (7). The clinical features of pharyngitis due to multiple different microbial pathogens are compared in Table 4.1.

Untreated Streptococcal pharyngitis generally resolves rapidly. About 75% of patients are afebrile within 72 hours after the onset of a sore throat, and the pharyngeal findings and tender cervical lymph nodes usually resolve a few days later. This relatively rapid response has made it difficult in some studies to demonstrate a significant advantage with treatment in terms of clinical response (8). Untreated patients usually show carriage of Streptococci in the pharynx for several months after spontaneous resolution of symptoms. With treatment, persistent carriage is noted in 6%–29% (9).

Table 4.1
Pharyngitis—Differential Diagnosis

	Pharyngeal findings				
	Erythema	Exudate	Ulcers	Cervical adenopathy	Miscellaneous features
Group A Streptococci	4+	4+ yellow	0	4+, tender	Soft palate petechiae Sudden onset
Group C and G Streptococci	3–4+	3–4+	0	3+, tender	Less serious No suppurative or nonsuppurative sequelae
Epstein-Barr virus	3+	4+ gray-white	0	2–3+	Splenomegaly Generalized lymphadenopathy Hard palate petechiae
Influenza	3+	0	0	0	Cough, constitutional symptoms
Adenovirus	3–4+	2+ follicular	0	2+	Conjunctivitis
Herpes simplex	2–3+	2+ gray-white	4+ palate	2+	Stomatitis
Enterovirus	2–3+	1+ follicular	3+ post palate	1–2+	Rash
Acute HIV	2–3+	0	2+ esophageal	2–3+	Splenomegaly Generalized lymphadenopathy Rash Weight loss

(continued)

Table 4.1 (continued)

| | Pharyngeal findings | | | | |
	Erythema	Exudate	Ulcers	Cervical adenopathy	Miscellaneous features
Mycoplasma pneumoniae	1–2+	0	0	±	Cough ± pneumonitis
Chlamydia pneumoniae	1–2+	0	0	0	Cough ± pneumonitis
Gonococcal	1–2+	1+	0	1–2+	Usually asymptomatic; history of oral exposure
Diphtheria	1–2+	4+ dirty-white	0	4+, tender	Exudate spreads over tonsils to adjacent areas; myocardiopathy and neuropathy
Vincent's angina	1–2+	4+ gray-brown	0	0	Putrid odor

Complications

Complications of Streptococcal pharyngitis are classified as suppurative or nonsuppurative. Suppurative complications usually involve adjacent anatomic sites and result in otitis, sinusitis, peritonsillar abscesses, and suppurative cervical adenitis. In rare cases involving highly virulent organisms, bacteremia with suppuration, such as pyogenic arthritis or osteomyelitis, is found at distant sites (10,11). These complications, which accounted for about 13% of hospitalizations in the prepenicillin era, have almost completely disappeared in recent years, presumably reflecting the extensive use of antibiotic therapy. A peritonsillar abscess is particularly important to recognize owing to the need for surgical intervention. This complication is usually not caused by group A Streptococci, but by a mixture of anaerobes from the pharyngeal flora (12). Clinical features of peritonsillar abscesses are an abrupt increase in pharyngeal pain, dysphagia, fever, and neck swelling. Inspection shows a peritonsillar fluctuant mass. Treatment consists of surgical drainage plus clindamycin. The nonsuppurative complications are summarized in Table 4.2.

Table 4.2
Complications of Streptococcal Pharyngitis

Complications	Comment
Scarlet fever	**Pathogenesis:** "Pyrogenic exotoxins" or "erythrogenic toxins" designated as serotypes A,B, and C cause the rash of scarlet fever.
	Presentation: Rash with tiny red papules (scarlatina rash), circumoral pallor, strawberry tongue (coated with red dots of

(continued)

Table 4.2 (continued)	
Complications	**Comment**
Scarlet fever (continued)	protruding papillae). Rash appears on day 1 or 2 of the sore throat, initially involves the face and then the trunk. Erythema resolves at 7–10 days and then there is desquamation especially of palms and soles. **Treatment:** Penicillin ×10 days **Second attacks:** Do not occur (prophylaxis not indicated)
Rheumatic fever	**Pathogenesis:** Frequency appears to reflect Streptococcal attack rates and prevalence of "rheumatogenic" M-protein types. Recent studies show that M-associated surface proteins of group A Streptococci determine both virulence and tropism (13–18). Virulent strains of M serotypes associated with rheumatic fever show an epitope (class I) that is distinguished from class II group A Streptococci associated with strains causing skin infection such as impetigo. Patients with rheumatic fever show serologic response to class I epitopes, but not to class II epitopes. The class I strains also contain epitopes that cross-react with host tissue and the N-amino terminal peptide of the M-protein has superantigen properties. The implication of these observations is that rheumatogenic strains of group A Streptococci show tropism for the pharynx, contain epitopes that presumably cause autoimmunity, and the superantigen property may be responsible for intense antigenicity.

(continued)

Table 4.2 (continued)

Complications	Comment
Rheumatic fever (continued)	**Presentation:** Jones criteria.[a] **Second attacks:** Common (prophylaxis indicated) **Treatment:** Penicillin ×10 days; salicylates or corticosteroids for symptomatic relief. **Prevention:** Treatment of Streptococci pharyngitis within 5 days of onset of symptoms prevents rheumatic fever. Recommended prophylactic regimens are: benzathine penicillin 1.2 mUI IM q 4 weeks (preferred); penicillin V 250 mg po bid; sulfadiazine 1g po qd; or erythromycin 250 mg po bid to adult or life (rheumatic fever) or to age 20 years and 5 years after last attack (rheumatic fever without carditis). **Duration of Prophylaxis:** to age 20 years and 5 years after last attack for rheumatic fever without carditis; longer for rheumatic fever with carditis.

[a]Jones Criteria from: Dajani AS, Bisno AL, Chung KJ, et al. Circulation 1988; 87:302. Prevention of rheumatic fever. A statement for health professionals by the Committee on Rheumatic Fever, Endocarditis, and Kawasaki Disease of the Council on Cardiovascular Disease in the Young, the American Heart Association. Evidence of preceding streptococcal infection plus two major criteria or one major and two minor criteria.

Major	Minor
Carditis	Arthralgias
Polyarthritis	Fever
Chorea	Laboratory findings
Erythema marginatum	Elevated acute phase reactants
Subcutaneous nodules	(ESR, C reactive protein)
	Prolonged P–R interval

Evidence of preceding Streptococcal infection: Positive throat culture or positive rapid Streptococcal antigen test *or* elevated or rising Streptococcal antibody titer.

(continued)

	Table 4.2 *(continued)*
Complications	**Comment**
Glomerulo- nephritis	**Pathogenesis:** Unknown; suspected mechanism is antigen-antibody complex or autoimmunity (19–22); restricted to few serotypes designated as "nephritogenic" strains—primarily with M serotypes 1–4, 12, 15, 49, 55, 56, 59, 60, and 61. **Presentation:** Proteinuria ± edema, oliguria and hematuria. Onset is 1–2 weeks after pharyngitis or 2–3 weeks after skin infection, but many are asymptomatic. **Second attacks:** Uncommon, presumably because the number of "nephritogenic" strains is limited or due to immunity (prophylaxis not indicated). **Treatment:** Antibiotic treatment has no established effect on the frequency or the course of nephritis. In epidemics involving nephrogenic strains, penicillin prophylaxis to susceptibles aborts the epidemic.
Toxic shock syndrome	**Prevention:** Role of penicillin treatment to prevent nephritis with *Streptococcal aureus* pharyngitis involving "nephritogenic strains" is not known. **Pathogenesis:** Pyrogenic exotoxin A or B that share biologic activity with toxic shock toxin of Staphylococcus (TSST-1) (23–25). The usual M serogroups are 1 and 3 (26). Streptococcal toxic shock syndrome is most common with soft tissue infections, although toxic shock with lethal outcome has been reported in an epidemic of streptococcal pharyngitis (27).

(continued)

Table 4.2 *(continued)*	

Complications	Comment
Toxic shock syndrome *(continued)*	**Presentation:** Group A Streptococci infection plus hypotension (systolic pressure <90 mm Hg) plus ≥ two of the following: creatinine ≥2mg/dL, platelet count <100,000/dL, liver function tests >2× upper limits of normal, adult respiratory distress syndrome, generalized macular rash that may desquamate (25). **Treatment:** Clindamycin often preferred over penicillin **Second attacks:** Rare or never

Diagnosis

The three methods used to detect group A Streptococci are throat cultures, antigen detection techniques, and serology.

THROAT CULTURE

Swabs should be obtained under direct visualization over the tonsils and posterior pharynx. This should be streaked on agar media as soon as possible. Various investigators have reported differing conclusions about both the incubation conditions and the optimal media (28–32), but most laboratories use sheep's blood agar with low dextrose content for incubation in 10% CO_2. Many technologists plant a bacitracin disk on the agar plate to facilitate detection of hemolytic Streptococci that are bacitracin susceptible. Carriage rates of group A Streptococci are usually reported at 1%–5%, but may be higher in epidemics, among children, and among adults with children in the household. This indicates a specificity for throat culture of about 95%–99%. Throat culture sensitivity has been studied with double swabs; these generally indicate a 9%–12% discordance

(33). In physicians' offices throat culture sensitivity may be substantially lower (34).

RAPID ANTIGEN DETECTION

The rapid antigen detection tests use either enzyme or acid extraction to remove group A carbohydrate from throat swabs followed by latex agglutination, coagglutination, or enzyme-linked immunoabsorbent assay procedures to demonstrate antigen-antibody complexes (35–39). Advantages of these tests include the immediately available results, cost reduction, and specificity that generally ranges from 95%–100%. The major problem is reduced sensitivity with reports ranging from 30%–95%. Reduced sensitivity is acceptable when Streptococcal pharyngitis is sporadic and the prevalence of rheumatic fever is low; a notable advantage is the potential for reducing antibiotic abuse with this type of screening.

ANTIBODY RESPONSE

The host antibody response is demonstrated with a fourfold rise in antistreptolysin O (ASLO), anti-DNAse B, or other antistreptococcal antibody titer, such as hyaluronidase, streptokinase, or NADase. Serology is the most definitive method to establish infection with group A Streptococci, but antibiotic treatment decreases the sensitivity. The increase in titer is generally rapid, suggesting a secondary amnestic response with levels greater than 300 U/mL during acute infection and peaks within 2–3 weeks. Serial rises in titer with sequential sera show titer rises of twofold or greater to ALSO or NADase in 80% of patients with Streptococcal pharyngitis (39). If two serologic tests are used, the increase is noted in 90%.

Based on these observations, Centor, et al. (40) have classified four types of Streptococcal throat infections.
1. Definite Streptococcal pharyngitis: Patient is symptomatic, and has both positive cultures and antibody response.

2. Possible Streptococcal pharyngitis: Patient is symptomatic and has positive cultures, but no antibody information is available.
3. Streptococcal carriage: Patient may be symptomatic or asymptomatic; have positive cultures and no host response; and positive cultures persist despite treatment.
4. Streptococcal colonization: Patient is asymptomatic and has positive cultures.

Management

Management strategies for patients with pharyngitis include throat culture, penicillin treatment, both, or neither. These strategies have been subjected to a frequently quoted cost analysis by Tomkins, et al. (41). These investigators used decision analysis with three strategies for penicillin therapy: *a)* treatment reserved for patients with positive throat culture; *b)* treatment of all patients, or *c)* treatment of no patients. Assumptions in the model included *a)* sensitivity of throat culture was 90%; *b)* the probability of acute rheumatic fever was 2.9% without treatment and 0.3% with penicillin treatment; *c)* the probability of dying or developing severe rheumatic heart disease within 6 years is 3.9% among those with acute rheumatic fever; *d)* the rate of serious penicillin reaction was 0.6% for parenteral penicillin and 0.25% for oral penicillin. Based on these assumptions, the authors recommended treatment of all patients with sore throats as most cost-effective when oral penicillin is used in the presence of an epidemic or when the probability of a Streptococcal infection based on clinical observation exceeds 20%. When the clinical features suggested a 5%–20% probability of Streptococcal infection, the most cost-effective strategy was throat culture with treatment restricted to those with positive cultures. When the clinical features indicated a probability of Streptococcal pharyngitis of less than 5%, the most cost-effective strategy was neither to culture nor to treat.

The Tompkins, et al. recommendations (41) require clinical correlations to define the probabilities of Streptococcal

---

Table 4.3
Management of Pharyngitis

MODEL 1: Discriminant analysis (42)
  Points for each degree of fever >36.1°C: +3/degree
    Recent exposure to Streptococcal infection: +17
    Recent cough: −7
    Pharyngeal exudate: +6
    Tender cervical adenopathy: +11

Total score	Probability of Streptococcal pharyngitis (%)	Management decision
−10 to 0	1.8	No culture; no treatment
+1 to 10	4.6	No culture; no treatment
+11 to 20	18	Culture, treat positives
+21 to 30	19	Culture, treat positives
+31 to 40	44	No culture; treat
>+41	100	No culture; treat

METHOD 2: Logistic regression (43)
  Indicators:
    Tonsillar exudates
    Tender cervical adenopathy
    Lack of cough
    Fever by history

No. positive	Probability of Streptococcal pharyngitis (%)	Management decision
0	2.5	No culture; no treatment
1	6.5	Culture; treat positives
2	15	Culture; treat positives
3	32	No culture; treat
4	56	No culture; treat

pharyngitis. This information has been provided with analyses by Cebul and Poses (8) using discriminant analysis and logistic regression. Clinical correlations with throat culture results in patients with pharyngitis show that the probability of positive cultures with each of the following: fever, exposure to Streptococcal infection, absence of cough, and presence of pharyngeal exudate. The decision is based on the presence or absence of these symptoms, with either point assignments for each observation or simply the sum total as is summarized in Table 4.3. For many clinicians, this approach provides a mathematical equation that equates to common sense. Thus, a patient with sore throat, coryza, cough, erythematous pharyngitis, and no fever almost certainly has a viral infection and does not need either culture or penicillin treatment. The patient with exudative pharyngitis with fever and cervical lymphadenopathy could be treated empirically for presumed Streptococcal pharyngitis. Cases between these extremes should have traditional management using culture with treatment based on culture results. An alternative strategy is to use the rapid antigen detection test for screening and treat those who have positive results. Owing to low sensitivity, culture is often necessary in patients with negative results.

ANTIBIOTIC TREATMENT

The four reasons to treat Streptococcal pharyngitis are to reduce the risks of rheumatic fever and suppurative complications, prevent the spread of group A Streptococci, and reduce the severity and duration of symptoms (Table 4.4).

Prevention of nonsuppurative complications. Classic studies from Warren Air Force Base in the early 1950s showed acute rheumatic fever developed in 2 of 798 (0.25%) penicillin-treated recruits compared with 17 of 804 (2.1%) untreated recruits (9). The rate of acute rheumatic fever in patients who had persistent Streptococ-

Table 4.4
Rationale for Treating Streptococcal Pharyngitis

Rationale	Comment
Reduction in rates of rheumatic fever	Studies in military recruits in the 1940s showed a rheumatic fever rate of 0.3% in treated patients compared with 2.1% in untreated patients (1,2,9,44).
Reduction in rates of suppurative complications	Parapharyngeal abscesses and suppurative cervical adenitis accounted for 13% of hospitalizations in prepenicillin era and now are rarely seen (9).
Reduce spread of group A Streptococci	Prevention of spread demonstrated with penicillin given both as treatment and prophylaxis (45,46). This benefit is implied by multiple studies showing eradication of pharyngeal carriage. Patients are considered noncontagious after treatment for 24 hours.
Reduction in severity and duration of symptoms	Early studies showed no apparent benefit with treatment in terms of duration of fever or sore throat (47,48). More recent studies have shown clinical response with early therapy (49–51).

cal infection despite antibiotic treatment was the same as it was for untreated patients (52). Further studies showed that 10 days of treatment was necessary for optimal rates of eradication of group A Streptococci; this could be achieved either with oral penicillin for 10 days or with a single injection of intramuscular penicillin G benzathine. Additional work showed that penicillin was highly effective in preventing rheumatic fever when treatment was delayed for up to 5 days after the inception of symptoms; a beneficial effect was also noted with treatment up to 9 days after the onset of symptoms (2,3). Since these classic studies, the rates of rheumatic fever in various parts of the world have shown substantial variation, and most developed countries now find this to be largely a disease only of historic interest (53). Rheumatic fever continues to be common in selected geographic areas including India, selected parts of Africa, the Middle East, and parts of South America (54,55). The cause of this dramatic decline in developed countries is not immediately clear. Poverty per se and malnutrition do not appear to play a decisive role because studies in military recruits fail to show this type of association. Some authorities feel this may reflect highly effective therapeutic intervention, but this seems unlikely when up to two thirds of cases occur in patients with asymptomatic Streptococcal carriage. An alternative hypothesis is a shift in epidemic strains. This hypothesis is supported by studies of strains in recent cases in the United States that show similarities with strains noted in the military epidemics in the 1940s and 1950s that belong to the notorious rheumatogenic M types (56).

Scarlet fever is another nonsuppurative complication that is found almost exclusively in children. This complication requires the production of erythrogenic toxins A, B, or C. It is another complication that was devastating in an earlier era but now has become a relatively minor complication (57).

Acute glomerulonephritis follows Streptococcal infections with only a few Streptococcal types referred to as "nephritogenic strains," which are distinctive from "rheumatogenic strains." With pharyngitis, nephritis is most frequent with M serotype, but nephritis frequency with this strain is only 10%–20%. Other nephritogenic strains are M serotypes 1–4, 15, 49, 55, 56, and 59–61. Unlike rheumatic fever, no convincing evidence shows that penicillin therapy prevents this complication, and recurrences of acute glomerulonephritis are rare, presumably because of the few serotypes that cause this complication.

Streptococcal toxic shock syndrome is a relatively rare complication of Streptococcal pharyngitis and is much more common with Streptococcal infections of soft tissue. Nevertheless, some case reports have been reported (58,59).

Prevention of suppurative complications. The second reason to treat Streptococcal pharyngitis is to prevent suppurative complications. The major recognized complications are peritonsillar abscesses and suppurative cervical adenitis. These complications, which were relatively common in the prepenicillin era, are rarely seen today (9,12).

Interruption of spread. A third reason for treatment is to prevent spread of group A Streptococci, which may cause epidemics or may be endemic. Transmission is common within families, day care centers, class rooms, and so forth. Transmission may be interrupted by penicillin therapy (45,46) as shown by multiple studies finding that penicillin, cephalosporins, and macrolides eradicate Streptococci from the throat of patients with Streptococcal pharyngitis. In general, patients are considered noncontagious after effective treatment for 24 hours.

Clinical response. The fourth reason for therapy is to reduce the severity and duration of symptoms, although early studies showed little apparent benefit from therapy, possibly reflecting the rapid resolution of symptoms in the natural history of this disease (47,48). More recent placebo-controlled studies have now shown a clear benefit to therapy in terms of clinical response (49–51).

Although a consensus currently exists that patients with Streptococcal pharyngitis should be treated, debate continues about the specific regimen. Group A Streptococcus, in contrast to *S. pneumoniae,* continues to be highly susceptible to penicillin with minimal inhibitory concentrations of 0.01 to 0.04 μg/mL. As noted, demonstrating a therapeutic response has been difficult so most efficacy studies are based on rates of group A Streptococci eradication from the pharynx. The assumption is that eradication from the pharynx correlates with risk reduction for acute rheumatic fever, suppurative complications, and transmission to contacts. Several studies have shown that penicillin treatment is optimal when penicillin V is given orally for at least 10 days or as a single dose of benzathine penicillin, 1.2 mIU intramuscularly (IM) (600,000 mIU IM for children weighing less than 60 lbs) (52,53,60,61). The goal is Streptococci eradication, which correlates with the prevention of acute rheumatic fever (50–52). Oral treatment for 5, 6, or 7 days is associated with streptococcal eradication rates of 50%, 77%, and 89%, respectively; the rate with a single injection of benzathine penicillin is 96% (61). Penicillin V in a dose of 1 g twice daily appears to be as effective as 500 mg given four times daily (62.) The problem with oral penicillin is compliance with the 10-day course, leading many to advocate the single parenteral dose. Most physicians now prefer oral treatment owing to the pain associated with parenteral injection, the need for physician or nurse time for injection, and the virtual elimination of rheumatic fever. Parenteral penicillin is still preferred when complications are likely and when compliance is predictably poor.

Penicillin has always been regarded as the drug of choice, and erythromycin (1 g/day for 10 days) has generally been advocated for those with penicillin allergy. More recently, the primary role of penicillin has been challenged by multiple studies indicating superior results with orally administered cephalosporins with two potential advantages: higher rates of eradication of group A Streptococci from the pharynx and a reduction in the duration of treatment necessary to achieve this goal (63). The higher eradication rates are unexplained because group A Streptococci continue to show susceptibility to penicillin at very low concentrations that are easily achieved in tissue with standard doses. A possible mechanism is betalactamase production by organisms in pharyngeal and tonsillar tissue, such as *Hemophilus influenzae, Staphylococcus aureus,* and anaerobes. Despite this observation, many authorities continue to conclude that penicillin is the preferred drug based on established efficacy in preventing rheumatic fever, its limited spectrum, and its low cost (64,65). With oral penicillin V, about 10% of patients continue harboring group A Streptococci, but these organisms are not important sources of pharyngitis in the host or contacts. Routine follow-up cultures and retreatment of carriers are not advocated except for patients with a history of rheumatic heart disease (65–69). As noted, the alternative for patients with penicillin allergy is erythromycin, such as erythromycin estolate in a dose of 1 g/day in 2–4 doses for 10 days. Acceptable alternatives include amoxicillin, oral cephalosporins, and clindamycin. Sulfonamides, trimethoprim, tetracycline, and chloramphenicol are considered unacceptable (65). Treatment should be started rapidly, but the delay imposed by waiting for culture results does not increase the risk of rheumatic fever (67). Treatment of asymptomatic carriers is not recommended except during epidemics.

A high prevalence of Streptococcal carriage by family members has been found (6,68), but not evidence showing that therapy is beneficial to asymptomatic carriers. Consequently, symptomatic members of the household should be evaluated, but routine culture and treatment of asymptomatic contacts is discouraged. Throat cultures to demonstrate eradication of Streptococci at treatment completion are not indicated unless rheumatic fever risk is high. The highest risk is previous rheumatic fever, es-

Table 4.5
Principles of Treatment of Streptococcal Pharyngitis

Treatment for 10 days is optional for eradication of group A Streptococci from the pharynx (1,2,4,53,60,61).

Treatment initiated up to 9 days after onset of symptoms is associated with prevention of rheumatic fever (3).

Early treatment significantly reduces the duration and severity of symptoms (49–51).

Penicillin, macrolides (erythromycin, clindamycin, clarithromycin, azithromycin), and oral cephalosporins have established efficacy for eliminating group A Streptococci from the pharynx.

The attack rate of rheumatic fever is the same in treated patients who fail to eliminate group A Streptococci compared with no treatment (52).

Throat culture at the termination of therapy is not indicated unless the risk of rheumatic fever is high.

Prophylactic treatment of family contacts is not justified (53).

About one third of rheumatic fever cases occur in patients with asymptomatic carriage of group A Streptococci; most patients with symptomatic pharyngitis do not seek physician consultation (69).

The risk of rheumatic fever is related to a prior history of rheumatic fever (especially rheumatic fever within 5 years or multiple bouts) and exposure to "rheumatogenic" strains of group A Streptococci.

pecially if it has occurred in the past year. Conclusions regarding therapy are summarized in Table 4.5.

Prevention

Avoidance of patients who have symptomatic Streptococcal pharyngitis is the major mechanism of prevention. The risk of transmission is notably decreased with treatment for 24 hours. Risk is also minimal for asymptomatic carriers compared with patients with symptomatic pharyngitis.

Tonsillectomy was once the most common major operation performed on children in the United States, most frequently for recurrent throat infections. This procedure is now relatively rare. It is generally reserved for a child who has at least seven documented throat infection episodes during the previous year that were characterized by fever, cervical adenopathy, exudate, or a positive culture for group A Streptococcus (70,71). Even then, the relative merits of surgery versus medical management are somewhat controversial.

For patients with rheumatic fever, the recommendation for prevention is penicillin prophylaxis, which should be continued for at least 5 years after the last attack of rheumatic fever **and** until the patient reaches his or her early 20s. Prophylaxis use beyond that period is determined individually according to the following risk factors:

- Risk increases with multiple prior attacks.
- Risk increases with selected types of exposures; for instance school teachers, parents of young children, health care workers, military recruits, and persons living in crowded conditions.
- The risk decreases with an increase in the interval since the last attack.
- A history of rheumatic carditis represents a risk for current carditis.

Regimens suggested by the Committee on Rheumatic Fever, Endocarditis, and Kawasaki Disease of the Council on Cardiovascular Disease in the Young of the American Heart Association for rheumatic fever prophylaxis are any one of the following (64):

1. Benzathine penicillin G, 1.2 mIU IM every 4 weeks
2. Penicillin V, 250 mg, orally twice a day
3. Sulfadiazine, 1.0 g, orally daily
4. For patients allergic to penicillin and sulfonamides, erythromycin, 250 mg, orally twice a day

References

1. Denny FW, Wannamaker LW, Brink WR, et al. Prevention of rheumatic fever: treatment of the preceding streptococcic infection. JAMA 1950;143:151–153.

2. Wannamaker LW, Rammelkamp CH Jr, Denny FW, et al. Prophylaxis of acute rheumatic fever by treatment of the preceding streptococcal infection with various amounts of depot penicillin. Am J Med 1951;10:673–695.

3. Catanzaro FJ, Stetson CA, Morris LJ, et al. Symposium on rheumatic fever and rheumatic heart disease. The role of the streptococcus in the pathogenesis of rheumatic fever. Am J Med 1954;17:749–756.

4. Breese BB. Treatment of beta hemolytic streptococcic infections in the home: relative value of available methods. JAMA 1953; 152:10–14.

5. Cornfield D, Hubbard JP. A four-year study of the occurrence of beta-hemolytic streptococci in 64 school children. N Engl J Med 1961;264:211–215.

6. James WES, Badger GF, Dingle JH. A study of illness in a group of Cleveland families. XIX. The epidemiology of the acquisition of group A streptococci and of associated illnesses. N Engl J Med 1960;262:687–694.

7. Poses RM, Cebul RD, Collins M, et al. The importance of disease prevalence in transporting clinical prediction rules: the case of Streptococcal pharyngitis. Ann Intern Med 1986;105:586–591.

8. Cebul RD, Poses RM. The comparative cost-effectiveness of statistical decision rules and experienced physicians in pharyngitis management. JAMA 1986;256:3353–3357.

9. Denny FW, Wannamaker LW, Brink WR, et al. Prevention of rheumatic fever: treatment of the preceding streptococcic infection. JAMA 1950;143:151–153.

10. Johnson DR, Stevens DL, Kaplan EL. Epidemiologic analysis of group A Streptococcal serotypes associated with severe systemic infections, rheumatic fever or uncomplicated pharyngitis. J Infect Dis 1992;166:374–382.

11. Talkington DF, Schwartz B, Black CM, et al. Association of phenotypic and genotypic characteristics of invasive Streptococcus pyogenes isolates with clinical components of Streptococcal toxic shock syndrome. Infect Immun 1993;61:3369–3374.

12. Mitchelmore IJ, Prior AJ, Montgomery PG, et al. Microbiological features and pathogenesis of peritonsillar abscesses. Eur J Clin Microbiol Infect Dis 1995;14:870–877.

13. Dale JB, Beachey EH. Sequence of myosin cross-reactive epitopes of streptococcal M protein. J Exp Med 1986;164:1785.

14. Bronze MS, Beachey EH, Dale JB. Protective and heart cross-reactive epitopes located within the NH$_2$ terminus of type 19 streptococcal M protein. J Exp Med 1988;167:1849.

15. Bessen D, Jones KF, Fischetti VA. Evidence for two distinct classes of streptococcal M-protein and their relationship to rheumatic fever. J Exp Med 1989;169:269.

16. Stollerman GH. Rheumatic fever: 1997 (Seminar Series). Lancet 1997;349 (in press).

17. Stollerman GH. The nature of rheumatogenic streptococci. Mount Sinai Journal of Medicine 1996;63:144.

18. Stollerman GH. Short analytical review. Rheumatogenic streptococci and autoimmunity. Clin Immunol Immunopath 1991;61:131–142.

19. Culpepper RM, Andreoli TE. The pathophysiology of the glomerulopathies. Adv Intern Med 1983;28:161.

20. Fillit H, Damle SP, Gregory JD, et al. Sera from patients with post-streptococcal glomerulonephritis contain antibodies to glomerular heparan sulfate proteoglycan. J Exp Med 1985;161:277.

21. Kraus W, Beachey EH. Renal autoimmune epitope of group A streptococci specified by M protein tetrapeptide Ile-Arg-Leu-Arg. Proc Natl Acad Sci USA 1988;85:4516.

22. Yoshizawa N, Oshima S, Sagel I, et al. Role of a streptococcal antigen in the pathogenesis of acute poststreptococcal glomerulonephritis. J Immunol 1992;148:3110.

23. Cone LA, Woodward DR, Schlievert PM, et al. Clinical and bacteriologic observations of a toxic shock-like syndrome due to *Streptococcus pyogenes*. N Engl J Med 1987;317:146–149.

24. Talkington DF, Schwartz B, Black CM, et al. Association of phenotypic and genotypic characteristics of invasive *Streptococcus pyogenes* isolates with clinical components of streptococcal toxic shock syndrome. Infect Immun 1993;61:3369–3374.

25. Working Group on Severe Streptococcal Infection. Defining the group A streptococcal toxic shock syndrome. JAMA 1993;269:390–391.

26. Musser JM, Gray BM, Schlievert PM, et al. *Streptococcus pyogenes* pharyngitic characterization of strains by multilocus enzyme genotype, M and T serotype, and pyrogenic exotoxin gene probing. J Clin Microbiol 1992;30:600–603.

27. Cockerill FR, MacDonald KL, Thompson RL, et al. An outbreak of invasive group A streptococcal disease associated with

high carriage rates of the invasive close among school-aged children. JAMA 1997;277:38–43.

28. Murray PR, Wold AD, Schreck CA, et al. Effects of selective media and atmosphere of incubation on the isolation of group A streptococci. J Clin Microbiol 1976;4:54–56.

29. Lauer BA, Reller LB, Mirrett S. Effect of atmosphere and duration of incubation on primary isolation of group A streptococci from throat cultures. J Clin Microbiol 1983;17:338–340.

30. Kurzynski TA, Van Holten CM. Evaluation of techniques for isolation of group A streptococci from throat cultures. J Clin Microbiol 1981;13:891–894.

31. Carlson JR, Merz WG, Hansen BE, et al. Improved recovery of group A beta-hemolytic streptococci with a new selective medium. J Clin Microbiol 1985;21:307–309.

32. Graham L, Meier FA, Centor RM, et al. The effect of media and conditions of cultivation on comparisons between latex agglutinations and culture detection of group A streptococci. J Clin Microbiol 1986;24:644–646.

33. Halfon ST, Davies AM, Kaplan O, et al. Primary prevention of rheumatic fever in Jerusalem school-children. II. Identification of beta-hemolytic streptococci. Isr J Med Sci 1968;4:809–814.

34. Rosenstein BJ, Markowitz M, Gordis L. Accuracy of throat cultures processed in physician's offices. J Pediatr 1970;76:606–609.

35. Otero JR, Reyes S, Noriega AR. Rapid diagnosis of group A streptococcal antigen extracted directly from swabs by an enzymatic procedure and used to detect pharyngitis. J Clin Microbiol 1983;18:318–320.

36. Knigge KM, Babb JL, Firca JR, et al. Enzyme immunoassay for the detection of group A streptococcal antigen. J Clin Microbiol 1984;20:735–741.

37. Meier FA, Howland J, Johnson J, et al. Effects of a rapid antigen test for group A Streptococcal pharyngitis on physician prescribing and antibiotic costs. Arch Intern Med 1990;150:1696-1700.

38. Wegner DL, Witte DL, Schrantz RD. Insensitivity of rapid antigen detection methods and single blood agar plate culture for diagnosing Streptococcal pharyngitis. JAMA 1992;267:695–697.

39. Stollerman GH, Lewis AJ, Schultz I, et al. Relationship of the immune response to group A streptococci to the course of acute, chronic and recurrent rheumatic fever. Am J Med 1956;20:163.

40. Centor RM, Meier RA, Dalton HP. Throat cultures and rapid tests for diagnosis of group A Streptococcal pharyngitis. Ann Intern Med 1986;105:892–899.

41. Tompkins RK, Burnes DC, Cable WE. An analysis of the cost-effectiveness of pharyngitis management and acute rheumatic fever prevention. Ann Intern Med 1977;86:481–492.

42. Walsh BT, Bookheim WW, Johnson RC, et al. Recognition of streptococcal pharyngitis in adults. Arch Intern Med 1975;135:1493–1497.

43. Centor RM, Witherspoon JM, Dalton HP, et al. The diagnosis of strep throat in an emergency room. Med Decis Making 1981;1:239–246.

44. Chamovitz R, Catanzaro FJ, Stetson CA, et al. Prevention of rheumatic fever by treatment of previous streptococci infections. I. Evaluation of benzathine G. N Engl J Med 1954;251:466–471.

45. Wannamaker LW, Denny FW, Perry WD, et al. The effect of penicillin prophylaxis on streptococcal disease rates and the carrier state. N Engl J Med 1953;249:1–7.

46. Poskanzer DC, Feldman HA, Beadenkopf WG, et al. Epidemiology of civilian streptococcal outbreaks before and after penicillin prophylaxis. Am J Public Health 1956;46:1513–1524.

47. Brink WR, Rammelkamp CH Jr, Denny FW, et al. Effect of penicillin and aureomycin on the natural course of streptococcal tonsillitis and pharyngitis. Am J Med 1951;10:300–308.

48. Merenstein JH, Rogers KD. Streptococcal pharyngitis: early treatment and management by nurse practitioners. JAMA 1974;227:1278–1282.

49. Nelson JD. The effect of penicillin therapy on the symptoms and signs of streptococcal pharyngitis. Pediatr Infect Dis 1984;3:10–13.

50. Krober MS, Bass JW, Michels GN. Streptococcal pharyngitis placebo controlled double-blind evaluation of clinical response to penicillin therapy. JAMA 1985;253:1271–1274.

51. Randolph MF, Gerber MA, DeMeo KK, et al. The effect of antibiotic therapy on the clinical course of streptococcal pharyngitis. J Pediatr 1985;106:870–875.

52. Catanzaro FJ, Rammelkamp CH, Chamovitz R. Prevention of rheumatic fever by treatment of streptococcal infections. II. Factors responsible for failures. N Engl J Med 1958;259:51–57.

53. Breese BB. Treatment of beta-hemolytic streptococci infections in the home: relative value of available methods. JAMA 1953;152:10–14.

54. McLaren MJ, Markowitz M, Gerber MA. Rheumatic heart disease in developing countries. The consequence of inadequate prevention. Ann Intern Med 1994;120:243.

55. Eisenberg MJ. Rheumatic heart disease in the developing world: prevalence, prevention and control. Eur Heart J 1993; 14:122.

56. Kaplan EL, Johnson DR, Cleary PP. Group A streptococcal serotypes isolated from patients and sibling contacts during the resurgence of rheumatic fever in the U.S. in the middle 1980s. J Infect Dis 1989;159:101.

57. Stollerman GH. The historic role of the Dick test. JAMA 1983; 250:22.

58. Herold AH. Group A beta-hemolytic streptococcal toxic shock from a mild pharyngitis. J Fam Pract 1990;31:549.

59. Chapnick CK, Graden JD, Leitwich LI, et al. Streptococcal toxic shock syndrome due to noninvasive pharyngitis. Clin Infect Dis 1992;14:1074.

60. Green JL, Ray SP, Charney E. Recurrence rate of streptococcal pharyngitis related to oral penicillin. J Pediatr 1969;75:292–294.

61. Mohler DN, Wallin DG, Dreyfus ED, et al. Studies in the home treatment of streptococcal disease. II. A comparison of the efficacy of oral administration of penicillin and intramuscular injection of benzathine penicillin in the treatment of streptococcal pharyngitis. N Engl J Med 1956;254:45–50.

62. Raz R, Elchanan G, Colodner R, et al. Penicillin V twice daily vs. four times daily in the treatment of Streptococcal pharyngitis. Infect Dis Clin Prac 1995;4:50–54.

63. Pichichero ME, Margolis PA. A comparison of cephalosporins and penicillins in the treatment of group A beta-hemolytic Streptococcal pharyngitis: a meta-analysis supporting the concept of microbial copathogenicity. Pediatr Infect Dis J 1991;10:275.

64. Dajani AS, Bisno AL, Chung KJ, et al. Prevention of rheumatic fever. A statement for health professionals by the Committee on Rheumatic Fever, Endocarditis, and Kawasaki Disease of the Council on Cardiovascular Disease in the Young, the American Heart Association. Circulation 1988;78:1082–1086.

65. Stollerman GH. Commentary: Penicillin therapy for Streptococcal pharyngitis—what have we learned in 50 years? Infect Dis Clin Prac 1995;4:54–57.

66. Bisno AL. The rise and fall (and rise?) of rheumatic fever. JAMA 1988;259:728–729.

67. Catanzaro FJ, Stetson CA, Morris AJ, et al. The role of the streptococcus in the pathogenens of rheumatic fever. Am J Med 1954;17:749.

68. Breese BB, Disney FA. Factors influencing the spread of beta hemolytic streptococcal infections within the family group. Pediatrics 1956;17:834–838.

69. Yalkenburg HA, Haverkorn MJ, Goslings WRO, et al. Streptococcal pharyngitis in patients not treated with penicillin. II. The attack rate of rheumatic fever and acute glomerulonephritis in patients not treated with penicillin. J Infect Dis 1971;124:348–358.

70. Paradise JL, Bluestone CD, Bachman RZ, et al. Efficacy of tonsillectomy for recurrent throat infection in severely affected children. N Engl J Med 1984;310:674–683.

71. Handley CO. Tonsillectomy: justified but not mandated in selected patients. N Engl J Med 1984;310:717–718.

CHAPTER 5

Sinusitis

John G. Bartlett

Snapshot Summary

Frequency: 1%–2% of common colds are complicated by suspected acute bacterial sinusitis.

Clinical features: Symptoms of a common cold that persist more than 1 week and include purulent nasal discharge ± headache, face pain, fever, and cough.

Diagnosis: Often based on clinical features.

Most definitive: Endoscopy and computed tomography (CT) scan.

Classification

Acute community-acquired bacterial sinusitis: "Acute sinusitis."

Nosocomial sinusitis: Secondary to nasal intubation; predominant pathogens are Gram-negative bacilli.

Chronic sinusitis: Symptoms longer than 8 weeks or more than four episodes per year of recurrent acute sinusitis lasting longer than 10 days.

Sinusitis in compromised host: Common expression of immunosuppression—common variable immunodeficiency, AIDS and so forth.

Fungal sinusitis: Noninvasive (most common), invasive (compromised host), and allergic (newly described form).

Bacteriology (acute community-acquired sinusitis):
  Sinus aspirates yield bacterial pathogens in about half.
    The predominant pathogens in all studies are
    Streptococcus pneumoniae and *Hemophilus.*
    influenzae (nontypable); less common are *Morax-*
    ella catarrhalis, Staphylococcus aureus, Strepto-
    coccal pyogenes, Gram-negative bacilli, and
    anaerobes.

Treatment
  Antibiotic selection: Therapeutic trials based on clinical
    outcome usually show nearly all antibacterials are
    therapeutically equivalent despite vase differences in
    in vitro activity versus anticipated pathogens.
  "Gold standard": Amoxicillin.
  Preferred agents based on in vitro activity vs. *S. pneu-*
    moniae and *H. influenzae:*
    Macrolides: Azithromycin and clarithromycin.
    Betalactams: Cefuroxime, cefpodoxime, cefprozil,
      amoxicillin-clavulanate.
    Fluoroquinolones: Levofloxacin, ofloxacin,
      sparfloxacin.
  Adjunctive therapy
    Drainage: Topical decongestants (ipratropium) or
      systemic decongestants (pseudoephedrine).
    Symptom relief: ASA, acetaminophen, ibuprofen.
    Allergic component: Topical corticosteroids and anti-
      histamines.
  Sinusitis is one of the most common clinical condi-
    tions encountered by primary care physicians and
    otolaryngologists. Current estimates are that this
    diagnosis accounts for about two million patient
    visits and 16 million prescriptions annually in the
    United States. There is good evidence that most
    colds are complicated by viral infections of the si-
    nuses, that about 1%–2% of colds are complicated
    by acute bacterial sinusitis and that the bacteriology

of these infections has not changed in the past 50 years. Nevertheless, sinusitis is the source of evolving management strategies with substantial controversies regarding management decisions including antibiotic usage.

Frequency

Studies by Gwaltney et al. using computerized tomography in patients with common cold symptoms lasting over 48 hours showed evidence of sinusitis in 87% (1). The implication is that the common cold is generally accompanied by viral sinusitis as well. It is important to emphasize that serial computed tomography (CT) scans showed resolution of the changes without antibiotic treatment. The term "acute sinusitis" has traditionally been restricted to patients with a specific symptom complex in which bacterial infection of the sinuses is either suspected or established. Using this more restricted definition, acute sinusitis complicates about 0.5%–2% of common colds (2,3). With an average of two to three colds per year in adults in the United States, this indicates about 10–15 million cases of suspected or established bacterial sinusitis per year complicating upper respiratory infections (URIs). There will be additional cases that occur as complications of allergic rhinitis and occasional cases ascribed to nasal obstruction, anatomical defects, dental disease or immunosuppression. The estimated number of cases of acute bacterial sinusitis is about 15–20 million per year in the United States and about 10% of these patients seek medical consultation resulting in approximately 2 million patient visits per year and the cost of nonprescription medications is estimated at approximately $3 billion per year (4).

Pathogenesis

The sinuses are normally sterile despite direct continuity with mucosal surfaces that harbor a rich flora (4,5). The pathogenesis of sinusitis is incompletely understood, but the assumption is that occlusion of the infundibulum is an important factor in predisposing to infection as is occlusion of draining orifices at other anatomical sites (1). Evidence for osteoinfundibular obstruction is supported by the CT scans during acute viral upper respiratory tract infections (1). Acute sinus infections are accompanied by inflammation and swelling of the mucosal lining with the accumulation of exudate containing acute polymorphonuclear cells in concentrations exceeding 5,000/mm. The extent of inflammation necessary for inclusion is indeed modest: for example, CT scans show the infundibulum draining the maxillary sinuses averages 6 mm in length with a diameter of only 3 mm. Drainage of sinus cavities is facilitated by cilia that move the mucous lining to achieve two to three exchanges per hour (4,6). The apparent source of bacteria with acute bacterial sinusitis is the flora of adjacent nasal passages. Nevertheless, the bacteriology of sinusitis is quite different than the normal flora in terms of the distribution of bacterial species. The bacterial flora of nasal passages is polymicrobial with large concentrations of anaerobes and streptococcal species. By contrast, acute bacterial sinusitis usually is monomicrobial with a very limited number of likely pathogens, the dominant pathogens being *Streptococcus pneumoniae* and *Hemophilus. influenzae*. Bacterial titers in exudates usually exceed 10^5/mL and may be substantially higher (4,5).

Clinical Presentation

Sinusitis is usually a complication of another condition that predisposes to this complication through infundibular edema with osteal drainage (Table 5.1).

Table 5.1
Predisposing Conditions for Sinusitis

Common	Uncommon
Upper respiratory infection (viral)	Trauma
Allergic rhinitis	Tumor
Anatomical abnormalities: deviated septum, polyps, and so forth	Foreign body
	Cystic fibrosis
Irritants—smoke, pollution	Primary cilia dyskinesia
Asthma	Choanal atresia
HIV infection	
Dental infection	
Nasal intubation or packing	

Acute bacterial sinusitis is usually a complication of the common cold and the symptoms of these conditions overlap extensively. The most common features are symptoms of a common cold that persist more than a week and include purulent nasal or postnasal drainage, face pressure or pain, headache, cough (from postnasal drainage) and nasal obstruction. Clinical features that have been suggested to specifically support the diagnosis of sinusitis include purulence of the nasal discharge, temperature exceeding 38°C and, especially, purulent drainage that persists over one week (4,7,8).

Physical examination usually shows purulent nasal discharge. With maxillary sinusitis, the pus is characteristically noted in the middle meatus. Transillumination usually shows reduced light transmission or no light transmission (5). Occasional patients have erythema or tenderness over the involved sinuses. An even smaller number show edema of the eye lids and excessive tearing suggesting ethmoid sinusitis. Fever is present in about half of patients with acute bacterial sinusitis.

Physical findings that suggest possible serious complications (Table 5.2) include *a)* chemosis, proptosis and/or limited extraocular eye movement indicating orbital extension, usually from ethmoidal sinusitis; *b)* meningismus, focal neurologic changes or altered mental status suggesting intracranial extension; and *c)* swelling, edema and tenderness of the forehead suggesting osteomyelitis of the frontal bone (Pott puffy tumor) (9).

Williams et al. (8) conducted a prospective comparison of 247 patients with symptoms suggesting acute sinusitis. The average duration of symptoms at the time of presentation was 11.5 days and the diagnosis of sinusitis was confirmed by radiograph in 95 patients (38%), most frequently maxillary sinusitis. Clinical features that predicted the probability of sinusitis by logistic regression analysis were: maxillary tooth ache, a history of discolored nasal discharge, poor response to nasal decongestants, abnormal transillumination and exam showing purulent nasal drainage. As

---

Table 5.2
Complications of Sinusitis

Central nervous system
    Subdural empyema (frontal sinusitis)
    Brain abscess (frontal sinusitis)
    Meningitis
    Cavernous sinus thrombosis or cortical
      vein thrombosis
Osteomyelitis
Orbit
    Orbital cellulitis (ethmoiditis)
    Subperiosteal abscess
    Orbital abscess
Respiratory tract
    Asthma
    Bronchitis

Table 5.3
Prediction of Sinusitis[a]

Symptoms and signs

Maxillary toothache
Colored nasal discharge by history
Poor response to nasal decongestants
Abnormal transillumination
Examination showing purulent nasal drainage

Probability of sinusitis

No. of predictors	Probability (%)
0	9
1	21
2	40
3	63
4	81
5	92

[a]Adapted from: Williams JW Jr, Simel OL, Roberts, et al. Clinical evaluation for sinusitis. Making the diagnosis by history and physical examination. Ann Intern Med 1992;117:705.

expected, the probability of sinusitis increased as the number of predictors increased (Table 5.3). Factors that did not predict sinusitis included painful chewing, fever, or sweats, ocular pruritus, face pain, headache, malaise, sneezing, sore throat, difficulty sleeping, or myalgias.

Classification

The major classifications of sinusitis are outlined in Table 5.4. They include:

• Community-acquired sinusitis: This classification represents the most common form and simply distinguishes

Table 5.4
Classification of Sinusitis

Location of acquisition

Community-acquired: usually seen with URI or allergy
Nosocomial: usually complicates nasal intubation

Duration of symptoms

Acute sinusitis: symptoms <6–8 wks
Subacute sinusitis: symptoms 6–8 to 12 wks
Chronic sinusitis: symptoms ≥12 wks or ≥4 episodes/year
  lasting >10 days

Microbial cause

Viral sinusitis: computed tomography scan evidence in
  87% of URIs
Bacterial sinusitis: complicates 0.5–2.0% of viral URIs
Fungal: rare cause of sinusitis

Host immune status

Immunocompetent
Immunodeficient:
  Hypogammaglobulinemia: congenital or acquired
  Compromised cell–mediated immunity: HIV/AIDS, lym-
    phoma, organ transplant recipient, corticosteroid therapy
  Chronic granulomatous disease

Non-infectious diseases

Foreign body	Midline granuloma
Nasal tumor	Cocaine abuse (intranasal)
Wegener's granulomatosis	

URI, upper respiratory infection.

community-acquired sinusitis from nosocomial sinusitis which has a unique pathogenesis and bacteriology
spectrum.
• Viral rhinosinusitis: As noted above, CT scans during a
  common cold show that most patients with an URI

have evidence of sinusitis, but there is no evidence of bacterial infection in more than 98%.

- Acute community-acquired bacterial sinusitis (ACABS): This is the form that most patients and physicians equate with "acute sinusitis," the implication being a secondary bacterial infection.
- Nosocomial sinusitis: This is a relatively unique form of sinusitis that has only recently been recognized. It occurs primarily in patients with nasotracheal intubation and the bacteriology is substantially different compared to community-acquired pneumonia; the predominant pathogens are *Pseudomonas. aeruginosa* and other Gram-negative bacteria (11).
- Chronic sinusitis: This is defined as sinusitis with persistent signs and symptoms of at least 8 weeks (some authorities use 12 weeks as the threshold) or four or more episodes annually of recurrent acute sinusitis, each lasting at least 10 days in association with persistent changes on CT scan for 4–6 weeks after medical treatment.
- Fungal sinusitis: A relatively unusual form of sinusitis involving a broad spectrum of fungal pathogens: Phycomyces (mucormycosis), Aspergillus, *Pseudallescheria boydii*, Bipolaris, Curvularia, Alternaria, and Cladosporium. These may be invasive, but invasion is found almost exclusively in the compromised host.
- Sinusitis in the compromised host: Patients with altered humoral or cell-mediated immunity are prone to high rates of sinusitis. The classic example of humoral defect is agammaglobulinemia (congenital or acquired, multiple myeloma, and so forth) with a high frequency of sinusitis due to *S. pneumoniae* and *H. influenzae* (type B strains). With compromised cell-mediated immunity, the classic example is AIDS. The problem with sinusitis in HIV-infected patients increases in terms of both frequency and refractoriness to treatment with progressive

immunosuppression. The pathogens in AIDS patients are not well characterized.

Predisposing Factors

Sinusitis allegedly effects up to 30 million Americans (12). Virtually all have predisposing factors that are summarized in Table 5.1. The most common, as discussed previously, is a viral respiratory tract infection, now sometimes referred to as "viral rhinosinusitis." The pathophysiologic mechanism, as summarized above, appears to be related to obstruction of the sinus ostium. Other conditions that predispose to sinusitis by a similar mechanism include allergic rhinitis and anatomical abnormalities such as a deviated septum or nasal polyposis, tumor, foreign body, and so forth. Another important factor is immunosuppression: sinusitis is probably the most common infectious complication of immunoglobulin deficiencies and it is extremely common with HIV infection (13). There is a well established but poorly understood association between sinusitis and asthma (14). It is estimated that 5%–10% of acute maxillary sinusitis originates from a dental source. This reflects the proximity of the maxillary sinuses to the molar and bicuspid roots with infection from direct extension.

Diagnostic Evaluation

HISTORY AND PHYSICAL EXAMINATION

Salient features in the history include the typical symptoms as described above with emphasis on the five factors considered to be particularly supportive of this diagnosis according to logistic regression analysis in patients with suspected sinusitis (see Table 5.3). Others who have dealt with sinusitis have distinguished major and minor criteria. Major criteria include purulent nasal discharge, purulent pharyngeal discharge and cough. Minor criteria include peri-orbital edema, headache, face pain, tooth pain, ear ache, sore throat, foul breath, wheezing and fever (15). Allergy as an underlying condition is suspect in patients with sneezing, ocular pruritus and characteristic exposures. With regard to physical examination, the expected finding is a purulent nasal discharge. With maxillary sinusitis there is often pus in the middle turbinate. Tenderness over the maxillary sinuses or frontal sinuses is helpful when present, but is not usually found. A minority of the patients have fever. Transillumination is useful in detecting sinusitis involving the maxillary and frontal sinuses. The exam should be performed in a completely dark room.

RADIOLOGY

The standard radiographic examination has been a Waters view that screens all sinuses. However, most authorities in the field feel that x-rays of sinuses are now antiquated by computed tomography that provides superior anatomical definition including examination of the extent of mucosal disease in the ostiomeatal complex (16). Deficiencies with plain x-rays of sinuses is well documented and is particularly problematic for ethmoid sinus disease. Prior studies of x-rays compared to sinoscopic findings have shown a good correlation in only about 50%, the major problem being false-positive x-rays (17,18). CT scan has subsequently become recognized as the "gold standard" (19). A concern about the relative merits of CT scan and x-rays is the expense of CT scans, although many radiology services now offer a four or five slice CT scan at a price comparable to routine x-rays. An additional issue concerns the indications for radiologic exams since 90% of cases can be diagnosed clinically with endoscopy. The most clearly defined indications for CT scan are:

1. Patients who are considered candidates for sinus surgery.

2. Acute sinusitis with suspected intracranial or intraorbital extension.
3. Patients with severe face pain or severe headache with unconfirmed sinusitis, especially if nasal endoscopy is not diagnostic.
4. Patients who fail to respond to standard therapy including antibiotic treatment.

Most otolaryngologists consider endoscopy to be the standard screening test prior to CT scan in patients with unconfirmed sinusitis (16). With regard to diagnostic accuracy of the CT scan, sensitivity is greater than 90%, but specificity may be relatively poor. Additionally, the demonstration of mucosal thickening does not distinguish viral and bacterial infection, although an air-fluid level usually indicates bacterial infection (4).

ENDOSCOPY

Endoscopy is often considered the preferred diagnostic method in terms of diagnostic accuracy and cost-effectiveness. This permits a detailed exam of the nasal cavity and the middle meatus. The correlation between CT scans and endoscopy for detection of sinusitis is usually 90% or greater (18,20–22). In some instances, endoscopy is more sensitive than CT scans (22). The exam is done with typical anesthesia and is well tolerated (23).

BACTERIOLOGIC STUDIES

The "gold standard" for microbial diagnosis is sinus-cavity samples obtained by puncture and aspiration (4). This should not be considered a routine clinical test, but is advocated in selected clinical cases and in therapeutic trials. The sinus puncture is relatively painless and safe when done by an experienced physician using a spring-loaded device. Maxillary sinuses are punctured below the inferior turbinate and the frontal sinuses are approached through the infraorbital rim. If there is no free fluid it may be necessary to inject saline. It is generally not possible to obtain uncontaminated specimens from the ostia via endoscopy due to the small diameter of the infundibulum and its acute angulation. Aspirate for culture are optimally done with quantitation with 10^4–10^5/mL as the threshold for "significant bacteria" (4,5) Alternatively, the specimen may be cultured by semi-quantitative techniques that are routine for most hospital laboratories; in this case, there should be at least five colonies in the second streak indicating "moderate or heavy growth."

Bacterial Pathogens

Among patients with suspected acute community-acquired bacterial sinusitis, only about 60% have verification of the presence of bacteria with cultures of sinus aspirates using the techniques noted above (4). Patients with high concentrations of bacteria also show high concentrations of polymorphonuclear leukocytes in sinus aspirates as well (5). The remainder are presumably ascribed to viral infections or represent infections involving organisms with fastidious growth requirements. The latter may include *Chlamydia pneumoniae* and *Mycoplasma pneumoniae*, neither of which have ever been detected in sinus aspirates but could conceivably represent a treatable cause.

The dominant bacteria in nearly all series using sinus puncture in acute sinusitis are *S. pneumoniae* and *H. influenzae* (4,5,24–28) (Table 5.5). Other bacteria that are occasionally implicated include anaerobic bacteria, *Moraxella catarrhalis*, *Staphylococcus aureus*, *S. pyogenes*, and Gram-negative bacteria. This tabulation of bacteria has not changed in 50 years, although there have been important changes in antibiotic susceptibility patterns.

Table 5.5
Microbiology of Community–Acquired Maxillary Sinusitis[a]

Viral agents (17)

Rhinovirus	15%
Influenza	5%
Parainfluenza	3%

Bacterial agents (4,5,17–22)

Agents	Mean	Range
Streptococcus pneumoniae	31%	20–35%
Hemophilus influenzae	21%	6–26%
Gram-negative bacilli	9%	0–24%
Anaerobes	6%	0–10%
Staphylococcus aureus	4%	0–8%
Staphylococcus pyogenes	2%	1–3%

[a]Adapted from: Gwalty JM Jr. Acute community-acquired sinusitis. Clin Infect Dis 1996; 23:1209. Results are provided for meta–analysis of multiple reports using sinus puncture and aspirates.

STREPTOCOCCUS PNEUMONIAE

This organism has always been the major identified pathogen in acute bacterial sinusitis. The pneumococcus was generally susceptible to multiple antibiotics and did not pose a problem for therapeutic decisions until recently. Since 1990, there has been increasing resistance to penicillin and to multiple other drugs as well. A recent review of 1527 clinically significant isolates are *S. pneumoniae* collected from 30 medical centers in the United States in 1994–1995 showed 24% were relatively insensitive to penicillin (29). Many of these strains were resistant to other antibiotics as well (Tables 5.6 and 5.7). This study included 52 sinus aspirates of which 20 (38%) were resistant to penicillin. *S. pneu-*

moniae is also acquiring resistance to multiple other antibiotics, especially the penicillin-resistant strains that show high rates of resistance to cephalosporins, trimethoprim-sulfamethoxazole, tetracycline, and macrolides (erythromycin, clarithromycin and azithromycin) (see Table 5.7). Fluoroquinolones, including ofloxacin, levofloxacin and sparfloxacin, are active against 99% of strains including 99% of the penicillin-resistant strains (30). Vancomycin is active against all strains of *S. pneumoniae*, but has the disadvantage of requiring parenteral administration and there is the obvious concern

Table 5.6
Streptococcus pneumoniae: **In Vitro Sensitivity Test Results with 1527 Clinically Significant Isolates Obtained from 30 Centers in 1994–95**[a]

Antibiotic	Resistant (%)	Antibiotic	MIC 90
Penicillin	23.6	Penicillin G	1
Intermediate	14.1	Ampicillin	2
High level	9.5	Amoxicillin–	1
Trimethoprim-	18	clavulanate	
sulfamethoxazole		Cefuroxime	1
Cefotaxime	3	Erythromycin	2
Ceftriaxone	5	Tetracycline	0.5
Cefuroxime	12	Cefpodoxime	2
Erythromycin	10	Cefuroxime	4
Clarithromycin	10	Cefprozil	8
Azithromycin	10	Cefixime	16
Chloramphenicol	4.3	Loracarbef	64
Tetracycline	7.5	Cefaclor	64
Vancomycin	0	Cephalexin	128

[a]Adapted from ref #29.

Table 5.7
Streptococcus pneumoniae: In Vitro Sensitivity Test Results with Isolates from 431 Patients with Invasive Pneumococcal Infections, Atlanta, 1994

Agent	Resistance (431 strains) (%)	Penicillin resistance (109 penicillin–resistant strains) (%)
Penicillin	25	—
Intermediate	18	—
High level	7	—
TMP–SMX	25	75
Erythromycin	15	41
Clarithromycin	14	41
Cefaclor	14	54
Cefotaxime	9	34
Tetracycline	8	24
Imipenem	6	23
Chloramphenicol	4	12
Ofloxacin	1	1
Vancomycin	0	0

regarding selection of vancomycin-resistant *Enterococcus faecium.*

HEMOPHILUS INFLUENZAE

This organism also ranks high on the list of pathogens found in sinus aspirates. The majority are non-typable strains. Treatment of *H. influenzae* is also somewhat problematic since about 20%–30% of strains produce betalactamase and are consequently resistant to penicillin, ampicillin and amoxicillin. However, most strains are susceptible to a large number of antibiotics including many that are frequently used in treatment of sinusitis such as second-generation cephalosporins, azithromycin, trimethoprim-sulfamethoxazole, tetracyclines, amoxicillin-clavulanate and fluoroquinolones.

MORAXELLA CATARRHALIS

This organism is now recognized as a pathogen with increasing frequency in sinusitis. Most strains produce beta-lactamase and are consequently resistant to penicillin and amoxicillin. However, this organism is generally susceptible to virtually all other antibiotics and consequently poses little problem for therapy.

ANAEROBIC BACTERIA

Anaerobes are the dominant components of the flora in the upper airways adjacent to sinus ostia and would be expected to play a relatively important role in these infections. Nevertheless, data supporting their role is checkered (4,31–33). The first major paper on the role of anaerobes in sinusitis was by Frederick and Braude in 1974 (32). Using specimens collected at Caldwell-Luk procedures, these investigators found anaerobes as the dominant flora in most cases of chronic sinusitis. There have been periodic studies examining this issue with variable results since that time (31,33). Most studies fail to use quantitative cultures that would clearly distinguish contaminants from pathogens, and those that have used quantitative cultures generally find relatively low concentrations. A prevalent impression is that anaerobic bacteria account for a relatively small portion of acute sinusitis cases and they play a controversial role in chronic sinusitis (4). The best confirmed cases are maxillary sinusitis associated with dental disease.

STAPHYLOCOCCUS AUREUS

This organism is found in the resident flora of the nose in 25%–40% of adults, but it is infrequently encountered in sinusitis aspirates. The yield with contaminated cultures using nasal, meatal or endoscopic aspirates is high.

GRAM-NEGATIVE BACTERIA

Pseudomonas aeruginosa and Enterobacteriaceae (*Klebsiella, Proteus,* Enterobacter, *E. coli*, Citrobacter, and so forth) are infrequently involved in sinusitis except in *a)* nosocomial sinusitis, *b)* sinusitis in the compromised host (primarily neutropenia and advanced AIDS), and *c)* with bacterial superinfections in patients who have had repeated courses of antibiotics.

Treatment

The goals of treatment are *a)* to eradicate bacteria from the sinuses; *b)* to prevent chronic sinusitis; *c)* to prevent central nervous system, orbital, and respiratory complications; and *d)* relieve symptoms. The usual therapy includes antibiotics selected empirically combined with nasal decongestants (4,34).

ANTIBIOTIC THERAPY

Antibiotics for sinusitis are divided into four categories (Table 5.8):

1. Historically correct: These are the drugs that have an established track record showing benefit. They include amoxicillin, doxycycline, and trimethoprim-sulfamethoxazole. Advantages are that there is substantial clinical experience, most patients respond and they are inexpensive—usually $9–$11 for a 10-day course at most pharmacies. The major disadvantage is that they are clearly inferior to multiple alternative agents based on in vitro activity against anticipated pathogens, especially *S. pneumoniae* and *H. influenzae*.

2. FDA-approved: These are the drugs that are approved by the FDA for the treatment of acute sinusitis based on clinical trial data. The group includes cefprozil, clarithromycin, loracarbef, cefuroxime, amoxicillin-clavulanate, and levofloxacin. FDA approval provides some physicians a level of comfort in a period fraught

Table 5.8
Antibiotics for Acute Sinusitis

Historically established

Amoxicillin	TMP–SMX
Doxycycline	

FDA-approved for sinusitis

Cefprozil	Cefuroxime
Clarithromycin	Amoxicillin–clavulanate
Loracarbef	Levofloxacin

Scientifically tested with pre– and post–treatment sinus aspirates showing pathogen eradication in >90%

Ampicillin/amoxicillin	Loracarbef
Bacampicillin	TMP–SMX
Cefuroxime	Levofloxacin
Amoxicillin–clavulanate	

Drugs with good in vitro activity

Macrolides	Fluoroquinolones
Clarithromycin	Ofloxacin
Azithromycin	Levofloxacin
Betalactams	Sparfloxacin
Cefuroxime	Ciprofloxacin
Cefpodoxime	
Cefprozil	
Amoxicillin–clavulanate	

with medical-legal issues, but many physicians and the FDA acknowledge that agents are commonly used with good justification despite the lack of an indication on the package insert. These drugs have the disadvantage of high cost, usually $60–$80 at most pharmacies for a 10-day supply.

3. Scientifically validated agents: Some authorities (4) feel that establishment of efficacy requires a pre- and post-treatment sinus aspirate with culture to demonstrate

eradication of the pathogen. These are hard studies to do, but when done, the success rate is usually 90%–100% with commonly used antibiotics (18). Antibiotics included in this category are trimethoprim-sulfamethoxazole, amoxicillin, amoxicillin-clavulanate, cefuroxime, cefpodoxime and levofloxacin. Advantages with this group is verified effectiveness with pre- and post-treatment cultures. A disadvantage is that many of these drugs were tested before there was a problem with penicillin- resistant *S. pneumoniae* or betalactamase-producing *H. influenzae.*

4. Modernized list of rational drugs by in vitro activity: This is a tabulation of drugs that are predictably active against most strains of *S. pneumoniae* and *H. influenzae* since these account for 75% of culture positive cases. Included are fluoroquinolones, macrolides (azithromycin and clarithromycin), amoxicillin-clavulanate and selected cephalosporins (cefpodoxime, cefprozil, cefuroxime).

It should be emphasized that several other factors are considered relevant in drug selection:

• Clinical trials: There is an apparent unexplained disassociation between clinical response in predicted response based on in vitro activity (Table 5.9) (35–40). For example, it has not been possible to show superior clinical benefit of any antibiotic compared to amoxicillin despite the presumed inactivity of amoxicillin against many strains of *H. influenzae* and *S. pneumoniae*. For example, Huck et al. (35) performed a randomized, double-blind trial of amoxicillin (500 mg three times daily [tid]) versus cefaclor (500 mg twice daily [bid]) in 108 adults with sinusitis. Sinus aspirates showed bacteria resistant to amoxicillin in 55% of recipients of this drug compared to only 10% resistant to cefaclor in that group; nevertheless, the clinical outcome in the two groups was comparable. Another trial

Table 5.9
Therapeutic Trials of Antibiotic Treatment of Acute Sinusitis

Reference	Regimen	No. Cured/ No. Tested
35	Cefaclor (500 mg bid ×10 days)	34/49 (69%)
	Amoxicillin (500 mg tid ×10 days)	33/47 (70%)
36	Penicillin V (1320 mg tid ×10 days)	34/41 (82%)
	Amoxicillin (500 mg tid ×10 days)	40/45 (89%)
	Placebo	25/44 (56%)*
37	Azithromycin (500 mg qd ×3 days)	174/221 (79%)
	Penicillin V (1.3 gm tid ×10 days)	163/217 (76%)
38	Clarithromycin (500 mg bid ×7–14 days)	50/55 (91%)
	Amoxicillin (500 mg tid ×7–14 days)	54/61 (89%)
39	Loracarbef (400 mg bid ×10 days)	165/168 (98%)[a]
	Doxycycline (100 mg qd ×10 days)	151/164 (92%)
40	Cefuroxime (250 mg bid)	98/115 (85%)
	Amoxicillin–clavulanate (500 mg tid)	102/124 (82%)
41	Amoxicillin (750 mg tid ×7 days)	87/108 (83%)
	Placebo	78/106 (77%)

*[a]Statistically significant difference for outcome based on clinical

showed 89% of 86 adults with acute sinusitis responded well to penicillin V (1320 mg tid) or amoxicillin (500 mg tid) compared to only 56% of 44 given placebo; this is one of the few studies to show antibiotic therapy was significantly better than placebo (36). Nevertheless, another recent trial in 214 patients with radiographically confirmed maxillary sinusitis showed no benefit with amoxicillin versus placebo (41). In one of the largest trials involving 438 participants, azithromycin (500 mg/day ×3 days) and penicillin V (1.3 gm tid ×10 days) were equally effective based on clinical response (37). These data suggest that antibiotics play a controversial role in acute bacterial sinusitis. It must be presumed that a large number respond without therapy (or despite wrong therapy) and these patients dilute clinical trials to the extent that it is hard to show differences. It seems likely that differences in clinical efficacy could be made with better patient selection, by inclusion of larger sample sizes or by meta-analysis. A challenge to those in this field is to identify the subset of patients who require antibiotic treatment (41).

- Cost: In a managed care era and with limited pharmacy plans there is continuous pressure to justify high cost antibiotics. The cost differential for most off-patent drugs (doxycycline, TMP-SMX, amoxicillin, erythromycin) compared to newer agents that have better in vitro activity (cephalosporins, amoxicillin-clavulanate, clarithromycin, fluoroquinolones) is $9–$11 compared with $60–$120 for a 10-day supply. It may be difficult to justify the use of expensive agents based on superior in vitro activity in the absence of data showing significant clinical benefit or cost-effectiveness.

- Compliance is a concern for outpatients medications. Prior studies show that compliance is improved with reduced daily doses so that once daily or twice daily regimens are desirable.

- Side effects must be considered. Associations that commonly limit usage are: TMP-SMX (rash), cefaclor (serum sickness), amoxicillin-clavulanate (500/125 mg formulation) (diarrhea), and sparfloxacin (photosensitivity).

ADJUNCTIVE THERAPY

Additional treatment considered important in improving outcome are facilitation of drainage and symptom relief.

- Drainage: The usual method to improve drainage is with anticholinergics (ipratropium—Atrovent), topical decongestants (oxyonetazone—Afrin, Dristan, NZT, and so forth) or systemic decongestants (pseudoephedrine or phenylpropanolamine). These agents presumably improve ostiomeatal and nasal obstruction, but serial CT scans show minimal impact on the rate of sinus drainage (4). Other methods to reduce inflammation are topical corticosteroids or antihistamines with anticholinergic activity. These have not shown impressive results except when allergy plays a significant role in the process.
- Symptom relief: Nonsteroidal anti-inflammatory agents, aspirin or acetaminophen are useful adjuncts for symptom relief.

Selected Categories of Sinusitis

NOSOCOMIAL SINUSITIS

Maxillary sinusitis was originally described as a complication of nasotracheal or nasogastric intubation in 1974 (42). The frequency of this complication among nasally intubated patients is 2.3% (43) to 96% (10,44) based on CT scan evidence of air fluid levels or opacification of maxillary sinuses. These studies have been criticized by the failure to detect pre-existing sinusitis and for failure to use adequate diagnostic criteria. One of the most definitive studies was by Rouby et al. (44) who excluded patients who had CT evidence of sinusitis and then randomized the remainder to nasal vs. oral intubation. Ninety-eight percent of the patients with nasal intubation had CT scan evidence of maxillary sinusitis and 38% of these had positive cultures with sinus aspirates. The dominant pathogens in this and other studies of nosocomial sinusitis were *P. aeruginosa, S. aureus,* and multiple coliforms (*E. coli,* Acinetobacter, *S. marcescens,* and *P. mirabilis*). This may be an important source of fever of undetermined origin in hospitalized patients. Recommended management strategies include CT scan for diagnosis, sinus puncture for bacteriology studies, antibiotic treatment, use of an alternative airway or gastrointestinal access source and, in some cases, surgical drainage (10,44).

CHRONIC SINUSITIS

This complication is defined as sinusitis persisting over 12 weeks or more than four episodes of sinusitis per year lasting more than 10 days with CT scan evidence of persistent infection despite antimicrobial treatment (45). The usual pathogenesis is ostiomeatal obstruction and the sinuses usually have bacterial colonization. The bacteriology is less well studied than acute sinusitis and results are inconsistent. Some patients harbor the same bacteria encountered in acute sinusitis (*S. pneumoniae* and *H. influenzae*), others have *S. aureus,* anaerobes and/or Gram-negative bacilli; some will show bacteria with low virulence potential including *S. epidermidis,* usually in low concentrations and of doubtful pathogenic significance (4). Polymicrobial infections are relatively common. The definition of the bacteriology of chronic sinusitis is confused, but also less relevant because antibiotic treatment plays a limited role except for acute exacerbations. Many of these patients benefit from surgery. Sinus surgery

was previously directed at sinus drainage e.g. Caldwell
Luc procedure, but this has now been largely supplanted
by endoscopic sinus surgery designed to correct ostiomeatal obstruction (4,45).

FUNGAL SINUSITIS

There are three types of fungal sinusitis:

1. Invasive disease that is usually seen in the immunocompromised host and generally caused by *Phycomyces*
   or *Aspergillus*. The course may be abrupt and rapid or
   slow and chronic. The infection tends to spread by direct invasion through bone causing osteomyelitis and,
   in many cases, intracranial or orbital involvement.
   Treatment often consists of high dose Amphotericin B
   and mutilating surgery (46).
2. Noninvasive fungal sinusitis is the form commonly seen
   in immunocompetent hosts and is characterized by
   sinus colonization without invasion. The most common
   fungal pathogen is *Aspergillus*, but numerous other
   fungi have been detected including *Pseudallescheria
   boydii*, Bipolaris, Drechslera, Curvularia, Alternaria,
   and Cladosporium. Nasal cultures will not distinguish
   invasive versus noninvasive disease; this requires
   histopathology (11).
3. Allergic fungal sinusitis was originally described in 1983
   by Katzenstein et al. (47). The disease is characterized by
   mucin secretion and inflammatory polypoid disease is a
   patient with a history of nasal allergy or asthma (48,49).
   The pathophysiology is thought to be IgE and immune
   complexes directed against the involved fungus. The
   major pathogen is aspergillus and this may have a pathophysiologic mechanism analogous to bronchoallergic
   aspergillosis. Other fungi implicated include Curvularia,
   Alternaria, and Bipolaris. Radiologic studies show involvement of multiple sinuses, and some have bony ero-
   sions. Inspissated dark mucus filling the sinus is a highly

characteristic feature at surgery; histology shows eosinophilic infiltrates and fungal hyphae. The usual treatment is surgical debridement (49).

References

1. Gwaltney JM Jr, Phillips CD, Miller RD, et al. Computed tomographic study of the common cold. N Engl J Med 1994;330:25.

2. Dingle JH, Badger GF, Jordan WS Jr. Illness in the home: a study of 24,000 illnesses in a group of Cleveland families. Cleveland, Ohio: The Press of Western Reserve University 1964;347.

3. Berg O, Carenfelt C, Rystedt G, et al. Occurrence of asymptomatic sinusitis in common cold and other acute ENT infections. Rhinology 1986;24:223.

4. Gwaltney JM Jr. Acute community-acquired sinusitis. Clin Infect Dis 1996;23:1209.

5. Evans FO, Sydnor JB, Moore WEC, et al. Sinusitis of maxillary antrum. N Engl J Med 1974;293:735.

6. Maran AGD, Lund VJ. Nasal physiology. In: Maran AGD, Lund VJ, eds. Clinical rhinology. New York: Thieme Medical Publishers, 1990;32–40.

7. Shapiro GG, Rachelefsky GS. Introduction and definition of sinusitis. J Allergy Clin Immunol 1992;90:417.

8. Williams JW Jr, Simel DL, Roberts L, et al. Clinical evaluation for sinusitis. Making the diagnosis by history and physical examination. Ann Intern Med 1992;117:705.

9. Wells RG, Sty JR, Landers AD. Radiological evaluation of Pott puffy tumor. JAMA 1986;266:1331.

10. Heffner JE. Nosocomial sinusitis. Am J Respir Crit Care Med 1994;150:608.

11. Washburn RG, Kennedy DW, Begley MG, et al. Chronic fungal sinusitis in apparently normal hosts. Medicine 1988;67:231.

12. NIH Data Book 1990. Bethesda, MD: U.S. Department of Health and Human Services; 1990:Table 44. Publication 90-1261.

13. Godofsky EW, Zinreich J, Armstrong M, et al. Sinusitis in HIV-infected patients: a clinical and radiographic review. Am J Med 1992;93:163.

14. Newman LJ, Platts-Mills TAE, Phillips CD, et al. Chronic sinusitis. Relationship of computed tomographic findings to allergy, asthma, and eosinophilia. JAMA 1994;271:363.

15. Shapiro GG, Rachelefsky GS. Introduction and definition of sinusitis. J Allergy Clin Immunol 1992;90:417.

16. Ziureich SJ. Paranasal sinus imaging. Otolaryng Head, Neck Surg 1990;103:863.

17. Pfleiderer A, Croft CB, Lloyd GAS. Antroscopy: its place in clinical practice. A comparison of antroscopic findings with radiographic appearances of the maxillary antrum. Clin Otolaryngol 1986;11:455.

18. Roberts DN, Hampal S, Lloyd GAS. The diagnosis of inflammatory sinonasal disease. J Laryngol Otol 1995;109:27.

19. Lazar RH, Younis RT. Comparison of plain radiographs, CT scans and intraoperative findings in children with chronic/recurrent sinusitis. Otolaryng Head Neck Surg 1990;103:183.

20. Kamal MD. Nasal endoscopy in chronic maxillary sinusitis. J Laryngol Otol 1989;103:275.

21. Nass RL, Holliday RA, Reede DL. Diagnosis of surgical sinusitis using nasal endoscopy and computerized tomography. Laryngoscope 1989;99:1158.

22. East CA, Annis JAD. Preoperative CT scanning for endoscopic sinus surgery: a rational approach. Clin Otolaryngol 1992;17:60.

23. Lanza DC, Kennedy DW. Current concepts in the surgical management of chronic and recurrent acute sinusitis. J Allergy Clin Immunol 1992;90:505.

24. Hamory BH, Sande MA, Sydnor A Jr, et al. Etiology and antimicrobial therapy of acute maxillary sinusitis. J Infect Dis 1979;139:197.

25. Gwaltney JM Jr, Scheld WM, Sande MA, et al. The microbial etiology and antimicrobial therapy of adults with acute community-acquired sinusitis: a fifteen-year experience at the University of Virginia and review of other selected studies. J Allerg Clin Immunol 1992;90:457.

26. Wald ER, Milmoe GJ, Bowen AD, et al. Acute maxillary sinusitis in children. N Engl J Med 1981;304:749.

27. Bjorkwall T. Bacteriologic examinations in maxillary sinusitis: bacterial flora of the maxillary antrum. Acta Otolaryngol 1950;83(Suppl):33.

28. Urdal K, Berdal P. The microbial flora in 81 cases of maxillary sinusitis. Acta Otolaryngol 1949;37:20.

29. Doern GV, Brueggemann A, Holley HP Jr, et al. Antimicrobial resistance of Streptococcus pneumoniae recovered from outpatients in the United States during winter months of 1994–95: results of a 30-center national surveillance study. Antimicrob Agents Chemother 1996;40:1208.

30. Hofmann J, Cetron MS, Farley MM, et al. The prevalence of drug resistant Streptococcus pneumoniae in Atlanta. N Engl J Med 1995;333:481.

31. Nord CE. The role of anaerobic bacteria in recurrent episodes of sinusitis and tonsillitis. Clin Infect Dis 1995;20:1512.

32. Frederick J, Braude AI. Anaerobic infection of the paranasal sinuses. N Engl J Med 1974;290:135.

33. Brook I. Bacteriologic features of chronic sinusitis in children. JAMA 1981;246:967.

34. Guarderas JC. Rhinitis and sinusitis: office management. Mayo Clin Proc 1996;71:882.

35. Huck W, Reed BD, Nelsen RW, et al. Cefaclor vs. amoxicillin in the treatment of acute, recurrent and chronic sinusitis. Arch Fam Med 1993;2:497.

36. Lindbaek M, Hjortdahl P, Johnsen UL. Randomized, double-blind placebo controlled trial of penicillin V and amoxicillin in treatment of acute sinus infections in adults. BMJ 1996;313:325.

37. Haye R, Lingaas E, Holvik HO, et al. Efficacy and safety of azithromycin vs. phenoxymethylpenicillin in the treatment of acute maxillary sinusitis. Eur J Clin Microbial Infect Dis 1996;15:849.

38. Calhour KH, Hohansen JA. Multicenter comparison of clarithromycin and amoxicillin in the treatment of acute maxillary sinusitis. Arch Fam Med 1993;2:837.

39. Scandinavian Study Group. Loracarbef versus doxycycline in the treatment of acute bacterial maxillary sinusitis. J Antimicrob Chemother 1993;31:949.

40. Camacho A, Cobo R, Otte J, et al. Clinical comparison of cefuroxime axetil and amoxicillin/clavulanate in the treatment of patients with acute bacterial maxillary sinusitis. Am J Med 1992;93:271.

41. Buchem FL, Knottnerus JA, Schrijnemaekers VJJ, et al. Primary-care-based randomised placebo-controlled trial of antibiotic treatment in acute maxillary sinusitis. Lancet 1997;349:683.

42. Ahrens JF, Lejeune FE, Webre DR. Maxillary sinusitis, a complication of nasotracheal intubation. Anesthesia 1974;40:466.

43. Grindlinger GA, Niehoff J, Hughes L, et al. Acute paranasal sinusitis related to nasotracheal intubation of head injuries. Crit Care Med 1987;15:214.

44. Rouby J-J, Laurent P, Gosnach M. Risk factors and clinical relevance of nosocomial maxillary sinusitis in the critically ill. Am J Respir Crit Care Med 1994;150:776.

45. Bolger WE, Kennedy DW. Changing concepts in chronic sinusitis. Hosp Pract 1992;27:20–22;26–28.

46. Morgan MA, Wilson WR, Neel H III, et al. Fungal sinusitis in healthy and immunocompromised individuals. Am J Clin Pathol 1984;82:597.

47. Katzenstein AL, Sale SR, Greenberger PA. Allergic aspergillus sinusitis: a newly recognized form of sinusitis. J Allergy Clin Immunol 1983;72:89.

48. Gourley DS, Whisman BA, Jorgensen NL, et al. Allergic bipolaris sinusitis: clinical and immunopathologic characteristics. J Allergy Clin Immunol 1990;85:583.

49. Berg NJ. Weekly clinicopathological exercises. N Engl J Med 1991;324:1423.

Index

Note: Page numbers in *italics* refer to figures; page numbers followed by *t* refer to tables.